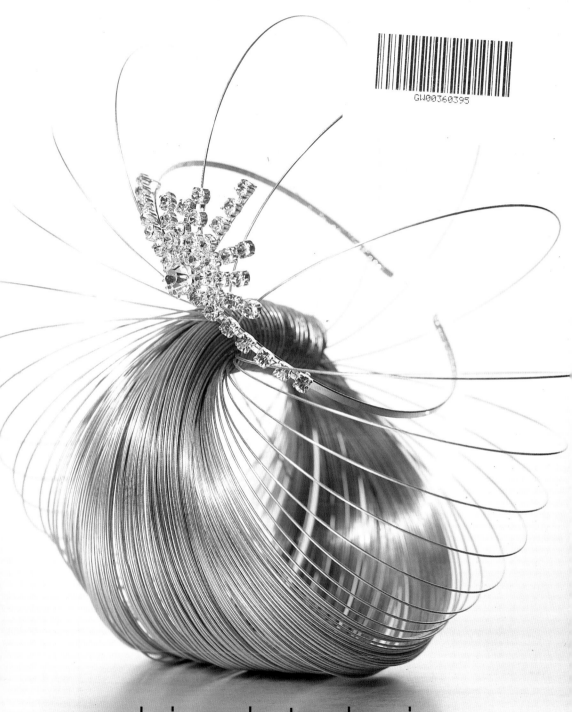

big date hair

THIS IS A CARLTON BOOK

Design, illustrations and photography copyright © 2000 Carlton Books Limited
Text copyright © 2000 Karen Wheeler
Original idea and concept copyright © 2000 Charles Worthington Limited

This edition was published by Carlton Books Limited in 2000
20 Mortimer Street
London W1T 3JW

A CIP catalogue record for this book is available from the British Library

ISBN paperback 1 84222 135 3
ISBN hardback 1 84222 217 1

The author, licensor and publisher have made every effort to ensure that all information is correct and
up to date at the time of publication. Neither the author, licensor or publisher can accept responsibility
for any accident, injury or damage that results from using the ideas, information or advice offered.

The application and quality of hair products and treatments, herbal preparations and essential oils is beyond
the control of the above parties, who cannot be held responsible for any problems resulting from their use.
Always follow the manufacturer's instructions and if in doubt, seek further advice.

Do not use herbal preparations or essential oils without prior consultation with a qualified practitioner or
medical doctor if you are pregnant, taking any form of medication, or if you suffer from oversensitive skin.
Half-doses of essential oils should always be used for children and the elderly.

No resemblance is intended to any person, living or dead, in the fiction element of this book.
The events and the characters who take part in them have no relation to actual events or living people.

Photographer (model): Hugh Arnold

Photographer (still life): Patrice de Villiers

Illustrator: Jason Brooks

Stylist: Sophie Kenningham

Make-up: Maggie Hunt and Chase Aston

Editorial Manager: Venetia Penfold

Art Director: Penny Stock

Senior Art Editor: Barbara Zuñiga

Project Editor: Zia Mattocks

Designer: Joanne Long

Production Manager: Garry Lewis

Printed and bound in Dubai

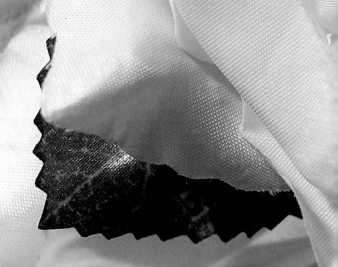

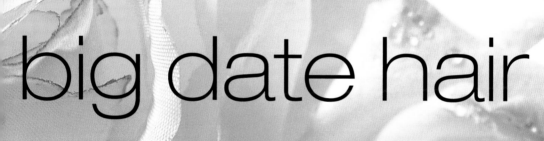

big date hair

Charles Worthington

with Karen Wheeler

CARLTON
BOOKS

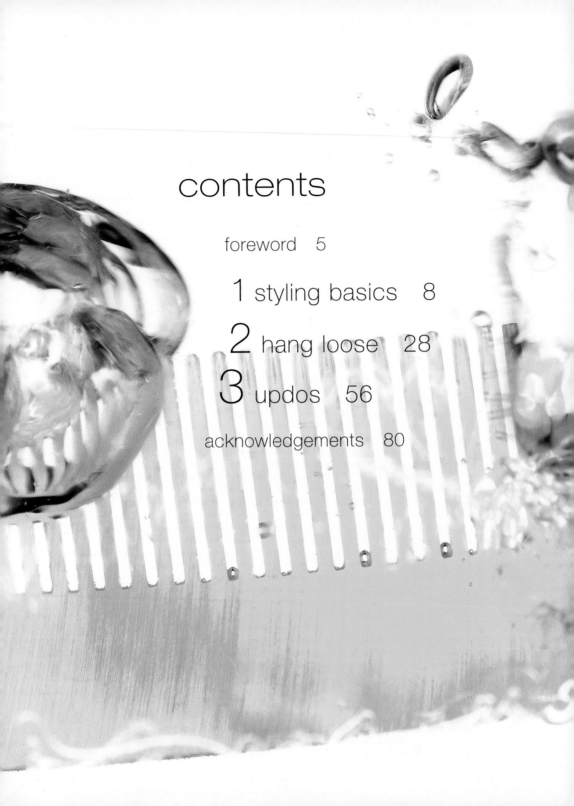

contents

foreword

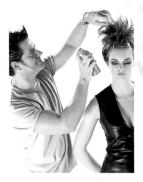

I know that some die-hard fashionistas may beg to differ, but never mind your choice of handbag when planning a night out, it's your hair that is your most important fashion accessory. Don't ever forget that your hair is the first thing that people notice about you. It speaks volumes about your personality, your lifestyle, your look and most of all, what sort of mood you're in: casual and laid-back, minimal and understated, glamorous and sexy, sleek and neat, or wild and va-va-voom? Glamourtime hair is also the most fun – there's nothing like transforming the way you look and feel with a blast of hairspray, a few pins and a bit of styling know-how. *Big Date Hair* is the ultimate feel-good experience. It covers your every hair need – whatever the invitation – whether you want to twist up your tresses in a ladylike updo to meet his parents for dinner or gutsy up your mane for a rock chick look that's got to last for as long as you do. Don't forget your faux-ponyskin handbag (OK, you do need that accessory, too), but make sure there's enough room for your hairspray!

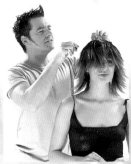

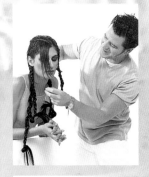

Charles Worthington

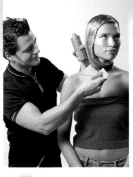

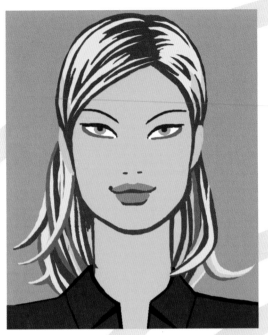

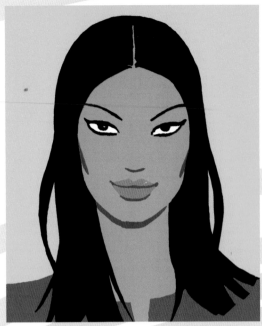

polly

Polly is a City career babe – traditional, yes, but she's got a twist. Her double first in maths means she can tot up her buying splurges as fast as the computers at Visa. A regular visitor to her Shepherd's Bush home is her boyfriend Harry – a good enough bloke but inclined to be insensitive; money is his aphrodisiac. Even he doesn't know that Polly's sleek blonde hair is the result of painstaking styling to iron out its natural wave. A flirtation with her American colleague, sexy cyber-suitor Simon, is giving Polly a new lease of life and looks.

jaz

Jaz (short for Jasmine) is your regular club bunnie. She loves all things hip, cool and girlie. Her earliest memory is of dressing up in the contents of her mother's over-stuffed wardrobe – and clothes are still her greatest passion. She can't remember the last time she took off her make-up before going to bed but, with her long, thick, glossy black hair, she always looks stunning nevertheless. Jaz has finally landed a job as fashion assistant at *Gloss* magazine, which has further fuelled her passion for fashion and new hairstyles.

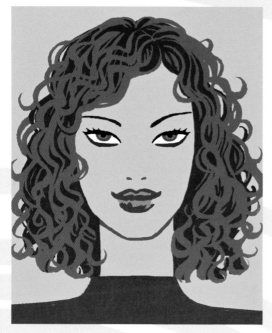

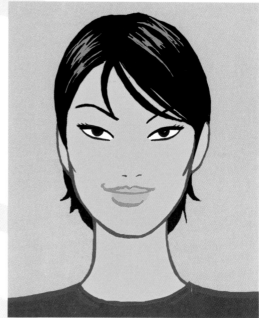

kate

Kate looks like a pre-Raphaelite painting: unruly curly titian hair, milky complexion and rosy cheeks. She works as a personal assistant to the marketing director of Crunch biscuits – not a good career choice when you have a sweet tooth and are prone to overindulgence. A hopeless romantic with an insatiable crush on her boss, Kate has decided that it's time to get ahead at work. She's convinced that a new, more streamlined image, complete with sleek 'power' hair, will help get her noticed – in more ways than one.

laura

Laura is a tomboy: lean and androgynous with a short crop. Her uniform is urban cool – more combats and trainers than pencil skirts and kitten heels. She loves to work out but is fiercely competitive and intimidates most of her fellow gym-goers. A struggling TV researcher who wants to make gritty documentaries and dreams of winning a BAFTA, Laura's recognized the benefits of networking. She's also trying to attract the attention of a certain assistant producer. Her redefined image – tomboy with a feminine twist – just might pay off.

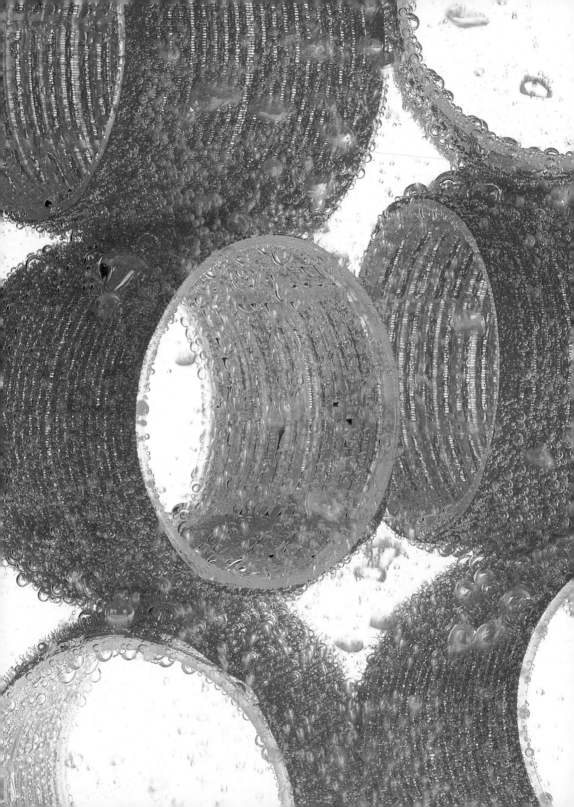

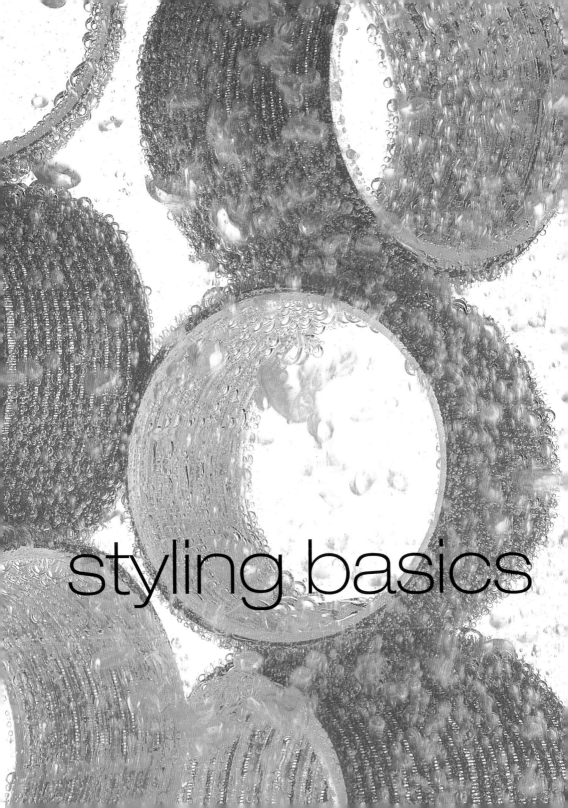

styling basics

the girls catch up

'So it was results all round,' said Chrissie with a self-satisfied smile as she retold the tale of the previous week's party at Shaft, the trendy new bar in Soho. The girls were sitting in Café Marron, their local coffee shop and favourite haunt, filling Polly in on all their news. Or rather, Chrissie was filling her in on their news while the other girls sat sipping their lattes, unable to get a word in edgeways. 'So Jaz got lucky on the job front; Laura was asked out on a date; and I've finally got my audition,' Chrissie recapped triumphantly.

Kate groaned inwardly to herself. Chrissie hadn't stopped banging on about her audition for this stupid new girl band, Pout, all week. Frankly, she was sick of it and it didn't help that she was so bored at work that she was now eating half-pound bags of caramel delights (misshapen and bought at staff discount) daily. It seemed that she, Kate, was destined to spend her days stuck in a dead-end secretarial job, piling on the pounds at Crunch Biscuits, while Chrissie led a fast, glamorous life. She tried to change the subject. 'So, Polly. How was your work trip?' Polly was stirring her cappuccino a little dreamily.
'What? Oh, um, fine, fine,' she said, turning pink and looking a bit flustered. If truth be told, Polly's thoughts were still in the Big Apple rather than in Café Marron. But she couldn't possibly tell the girls about her little moment of passion with Simon, her sexy American colleague. She blushed again as she remembered the long, lingering kiss …

Her flatmates eyed her suspiciously. For someone who had stepped off an overnight flight from New York just a few hours earlier, Polly was looking intriguingly good. Her skin was glowing, her hair looked fashionably dishevelled (as opposed to City-girl neat) and she was wearing stiletto boots with a pair of new, tight, bootleg jeans (bought in SoHo). Polly, sensible Polly, was looking rather foxy.
'So did you miss Harry dreadfully?' Kate persisted.
'Harry?' said Polly.
'You know, your boyfriend,' quipped Laura, sarcastically.

Fortunately, Polly was saved from answering by Chrissie's burning dilemma. 'I simply can't decide what to wear for my audition,' she was saying. 'It's a toss-up between my lucky red dress – the strapless one – and my snakeskin-print jeans. Jaz, maybe you could style me?' Jaz had been practically bouncing up and down with excitement for the past half hour (and it wasn't the effect of the caffeine).
'Oh, I'd love to. I start my work placement at *Gloss* on Monday, so maybe I'll be able to borrow a designer outfit for you to wear.'

Polly's ears pricked up. 'Work placement? But Jaz, what about your job at The Flag? You do know that a work placement means you don't get paid, don't you?'
'*Gloss* is going to pay my travel expenses,' said Jaz, hugging her fuchsia fishnetted knees with excitement. Laura – who had long thought that Jaz came from a completely different planet – stifled a snigger.
'Only travel expenses? How are you going to pay your rent?' asked Polly, dragged back suddenly from her daydream. She was, after all, Jaz's landlady.
'Oh, I'll get an evening job in a bar or something,' said Jaz, her eyes shining at the thought of meeting the world's top fashion designers and models, and travelling across the globe on *Gloss* fashion shoots.

Polly sighed. Life at 23 Havana Road, Shepherds Bush was certainly going to be interesting in the next few weeks. Not least, she thought with a pang of guilt, because sexy Simon had promised to call.

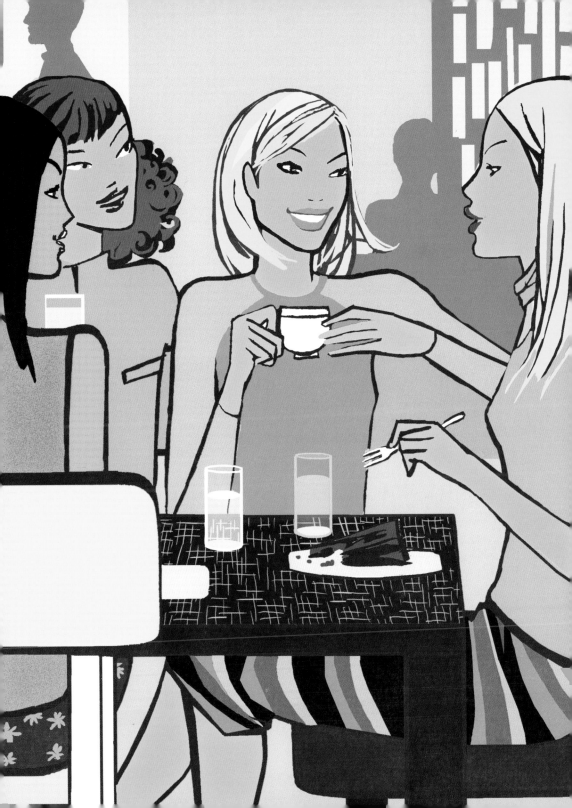

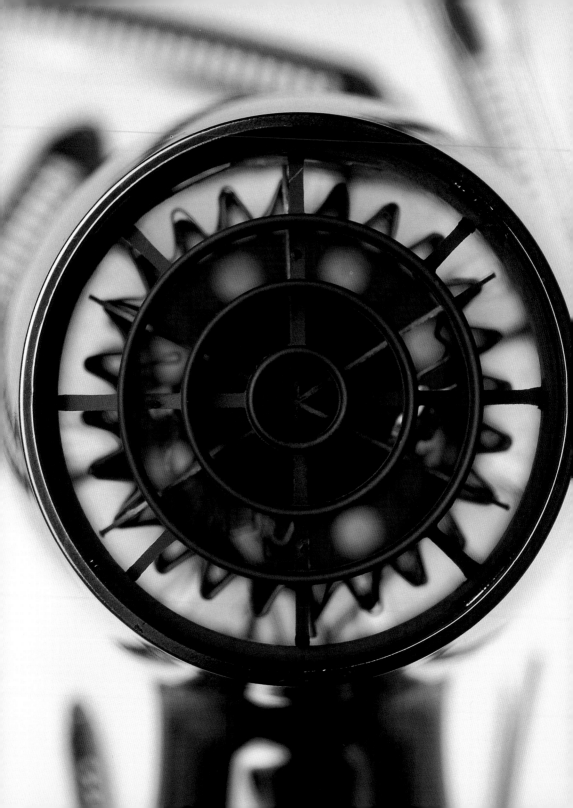

stylist's tool box

You don't need a new haircut or a visit to the salon to achieve wow-factor hair. With a little know-how and the right tools you can perform mini miracles at home. Girls born without curls, for example, can win the battle against nature and give themselves Julia Roberts'-style corkscrews. Similarly, those who are blessed (or cursed, depending on your point of view) with a surfeit of kinks and curls, can make their hair stick-straight, simply by using the right styling products and drying technique. Hair is the ultimate fashion accessory. The golden rule is that if it looks good, you'll feel good. Here's what the professionals have in their tool box:

the gadgets

hairdryer

Not just for blasting wet hair dry, a hairdryer can make your hair sleek and straight, or give it more lift than a pair of Manolos. Make sure yours is at least 1,500 watts, otherwise you will spend valuable date time drying your hair and possibly even damage it in the process.

diffuser

This big, dish-like attachment is used to dry curly hair. It disperses the flow of air so that curls, natural or otherwise, aren't straightened by its sheer force.

brushes

Styling is about shaping the hair, so don't think you can use the same brush as for everyday grooming. Styling brushes come in many shapes and sizes. Flat brushes, which have bristles on one side only, are good, all-round tools, but are not precise enough to curl or straighten the hair. Round brushes, with bristles all the way around, are for curling, straightening or adding volume. Use small-diameter brushes for short hair and large-diameter ones for straightening kinks out of long hair. Broad, flat paddle brushes are great for blow-drying straight or wavy long hair, as well as for styling hair to a poker-straight finish.

combs

You need a good, all-purpose comb for detangling hair, dividing it into sections and for backcombing.

curling tongs

These create curls for girls who don't have them. Use small-diameter tongs for short hair or for making tight curls, and large tongs for creating looser curls in long hair. You can also get heated curling brushes, which have bristles rather than a clamp to hold the hair in place. Use tongs on dry hair only.

straightening irons

These are used after blow-drying to give a blunt, poker straight look. The two flat, heated plates are clamped over a section of hair and slowly drawn down to the ends. They should not be used too often as they are very dehydrating.

crimping irons

As well as creating the distinctive 'corrugated' wave that goes in and out of fashion faster than flared trousers, these irons can also be used on the under layers of dry hair to boost volume, or at the roots to lift limp hair.

rollers

Rollers, which can be used to add volume to hair as well as make it curly, have become very hip. And hurrah for the fact that – unlike your grandmother's generation – you don't have to go to bed wearing them. Heated rollers (for use on dry hair only) are a speedy way of creating strong curls. For loose curls, take out the rollers while they are still warm. Velcro rollers are non-heated but you can put them into dry or damp hair to add lift at the roots.

hairpins, grips and sectioning clips

Small hairpins and grips are essential for securing updos and small sections of hair – use matt ones, which are less slippery, in a colour that matches your hair. Big metal clips are useful when you need to hold larger sections of hair up and out of the way for styling.

Chrissie is leaving nothing to chance. Tomorrow is her big audition with Pout, so she's locked herself in the bathroom for yet another experiment. She knows it's going to annoy Kate, who's already started to make snide comments about Chrissie hogging the bathroom all the time, but it just can't be helped. Chrissie's determined to turn her fine blonde hair into big hair and the way to do it, she's read in one of her many beauty books, is to use extra-large rollers. Standing in front of the bathroom mirror, she finishes rolling the last big Velcro roller

... chrissie tries big hair for size

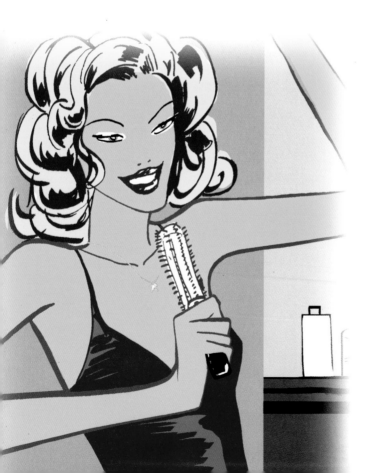

snugly against her scalp (for maximum volume) and spritzes her hair with styling spray. Ten minutes later Chrissie carefully removes the rollers and admires herself with a satisfied (almost smug – Laura would call it narcissistic) smile. Not only does her hair look bigger and bouncier, but the strapless red dress shows off her fake tan to perfection. Jaz has tried to convince her to wear her python-print jeans and a pussy-cat bow blouse, but Chrissie knows better. The other girls from Pout practically live in snakeskin-print jeans, and she wants to look different. In her tight scarlet dress (holding her hairbrush to her mouth in mock singing/karaoke mode) and with her limp blonde locks transformed into big voluminous hair, there is no doubt that Chrissie is going to stand out from the crowd ...

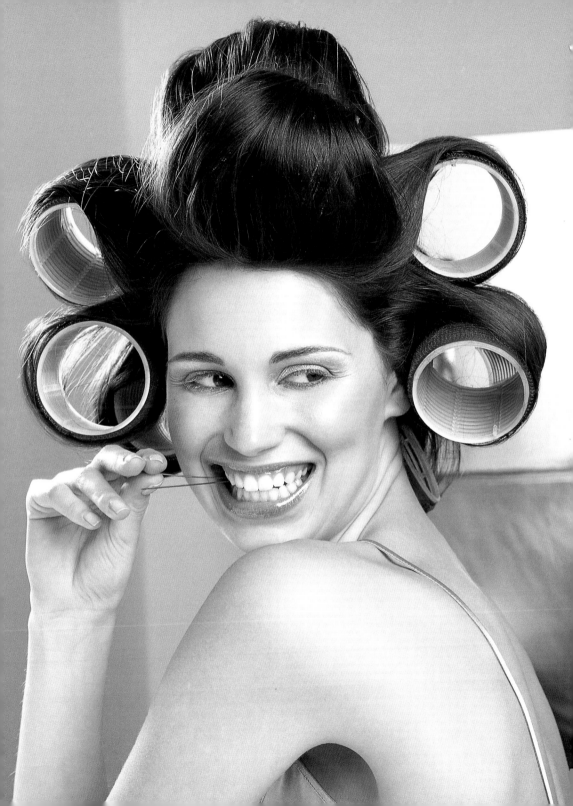

the products

If you don't know a serum from a shine spray, the range of styling lotions and potions out there is enough to make your hair curl. But you don't need a whole battery of products: the contents of your personal tool box will depend on your particular hair type and the style that you want to achieve.

wax and pomade

Wax and pomade are designed to add definition and hold. They come in numerous strengths, holds and consistencies, so it might take a while to find the best one for you – but once you've found it, you won't ever want to be without it.

anti-frizz serum

This is the product for eliminating frizzy, flyaway bits and for bringing unruly hair to heel. It contains silicone, which coats the hair shaft and smooths and seals the cuticle. Use it on wet hair before styling or to smooth down dry hair. Serum can be mixed with other products to give extra-glossy drying and extra protection.

curl revitalizer and activator

These perk up deflated curls by adding moisture – but only if the curl existed in the first place. These products tend to come in gel form, and the more product used, the more defined the curl. Test these products before a big night out, as too much can sometimes overload the hair.

styling cream

Similar to leave-in conditioner, this acts as a form of damage limitation if you apply it to the ends of the hair before using heated appliances. Volume control or non-chemical relaxers normally come in a cream form and should be used sparingly.

shine enhancer

This usually comes in spray or liquid form and contains silicone to coat the hair shaft, smooth the cuticle and add the magic shine factor. Shine spray is an absolute must-have for perfect, glossy, glamour hair.

mousse

A light and airy foam that is used to add oomph to fine hair (apply it to the roots before blow-drying) or to shape and control dry hair. Mousse comes in varying strengths and can be used for softer setting techniques.

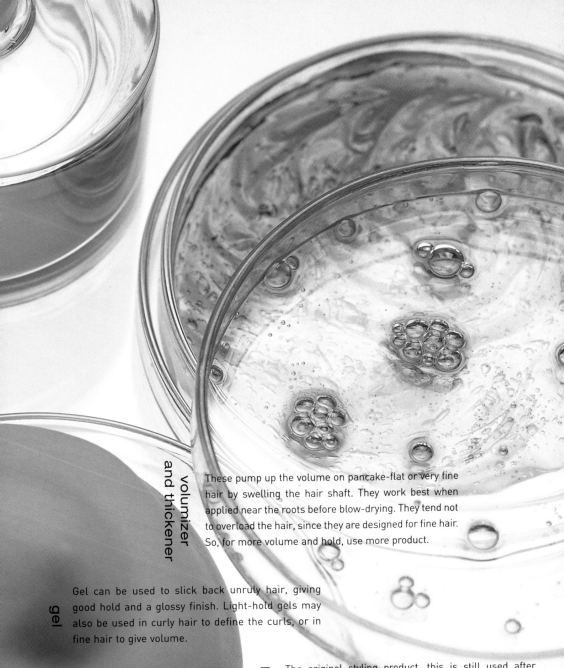

volumizer and thickener

These pump up the volume on pancake-flat or very fine hair by swelling the hair shaft. They work best when applied near the roots before blow-drying. They tend not to overload the hair, since they are designed for fine hair. So, for more volume and hold, use more product.

gel

Gel can be used to slick back unruly hair, giving good hold and a glossy finish. Light-hold gels may also be used in curly hair to define the curls, or in fine hair to give volume.

hairspray

The original styling product, this is still used after styling to hold hair in place. Useful for updos and styles that need to keep their shape. Hairsprays come in different strengths, so choose one for your desired hold. Hairspray also helps to reduce static.

back to basics

Before you launch into the groovy world of transforming your tresses with rollers, plaits and updos, there are a few fundamental styling techniques that are essential to master for the best results.

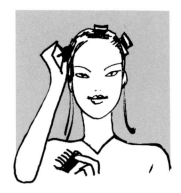

sleek hair

you need

Blow-drying spray • sectioning clips • large straightening brush (a paddle brush is ideal) • hairdryer • straightening irons • serum

1 Shampoo and towel-dry your hair, then cover it evenly in a light mist of blow-drying spray.

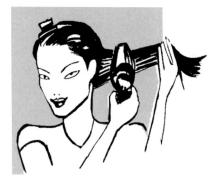

2 Starting at the back and working forwards, section off the hair with big clips. Using a large straightening brush, starting at the roots, point the hairdryer nozzle downwards and move it down a small section of hair at the same time as the brush.

3 Once you have finished drying each section, switch the hairdryer to the cold setting as this will close the cuticles and leave the hair glossier.

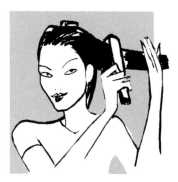

4 Heat the straightening irons until they are hot and run them from the roots to the ends of the hair. This will seal the cuticles, leaving it almost impossible for any moisture to penetrate the hair shaft.

HAIR SNIP

FOR A SUPER-GLOSSY FINISH, RUB A SMALL AMOUNT OF SERUM IN THE PALM OF ONE HAND AND SMOOTH IT OVER THE SURFACE OF YOUR HAIR TO FLATTEN DOWN ANY STRAY WISPS.

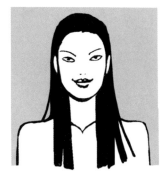

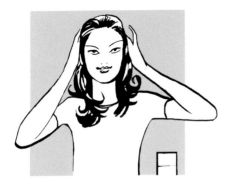

great curls

you need

Styling product suitable for your hair type (some mousses or volumizers help to boost curl and make the whole styling and drying process much easier) • hairdryer and diffuser • shine spray • serum

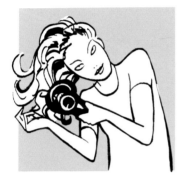

1 After shampooing and conditioning the hair, blot it gently with a towel to absorb as much moisture as possible. Be especially careful not to rub curly hair as this roughs up the cuticle and causes the hair to frizz and look dull.

2 Apply your chosen styling product, distributing it evenly over the hair – it is really important to start with a great foundation.

3 Tip your head to one side and, using the bowl of the diffuser, lift the hairdryer up and down into the hair with a gentle movement. Then tip your head to the other side and repeat.

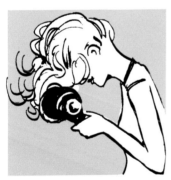

4 When the hair is dry, tip your head forward and carry on with a similar motion. If you find your hair is starting to go fluffy, spritz it with a shine spray.

5 When you have finished drying all of the hair in this way, gently run a small amount of serum evenly through it to create a more defined curl.

HAIR SNIP

YOU MAY FIND THAT A DAY OR TWO AFTER YOU'VE WASHED AND BLOW-DRIED YOUR HAIR, SECTIONS MAY START TO BECOME FRIZZY AND TANGLED. IF THIS IS THE CASE, SIMPLY SPRITZ YOUR HAIR WITH WATER USING A PLANT MISTER AND PULL YOUR FINGERS THROUGH IT GENTLY TO SEPARATE AND DEFINE THE CURLS. THEN LET IT DRY NATURALLY. HANDLING YOUR HAIR AS LITTLE AS POSSIBLE WILL HELP PREVENT FRIZZINESS.

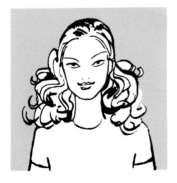

big hair

you need

Hairdryer • volumizing
mousse or blow-
drying spray •
sectioning clips •
brush with a
detachable bristle
roller • hairspray

1 After shampooing and
conditioning, blow-dry the hair
roughly until it is 70 per cent dry.

2 Evenly apply the mousse or blow-drying spray.

3 Pin up the top layer of the hair so that you
can access the layer underneath. Dry it section
by section, using the roller brush to hold the roots
at right angles to the scalp as you do so.

4 Unclip the top layer section by section and dry
each one in the same way, this time unclipping the
handle of the brush and leaving the roller in the hair
to set in volume. This creates a soft fullness that lifts
the hair away from the head. It also smooths and
softens the hair cuticles, maximizing gloss and shine.

5 Give the hair a blast of cold air, then remove
the brush head once the hair is completely cool.

6 When you have finished drying all the hair, shape
it with your fingers and lightly spritz with hairspray.

textured hair

you need

Medium-hold gel • comb • hairdryer

1 A quick, easy way of adding texture to hair of any
length is to apply a little medium-hold gel to the root
area. You can do this on wet hair or dry hair.

2 Comb the gel through the hair and then,
using a warm setting on the hairdryer, direct
the heat at the roots and use your fingers to
lift the hair as you do so.

3 Once the roots are dry,
take the heat through to the
ends of your hair, combing
it with your fingers. This
gives a slightly messy
and windblown look.

4 For ultimate 'rock
chick' texture and great
volume, finish by tipping
your head upside-down
and gently roughing up
the hair with your hands.

styling secrets for those
in the know

Always finish blow-drying your hair with a quick blast
of cold air. Not only does it 'set' the new shape in
place, but it closes the hair cuticles which maximizes
gloss and shine. (When the cuticles lie flat, they
reflect the light better.) Now that's a cute tip!

For best blow-drying results, gently dry the hair
until it is 70 per cent dry before attempting to style
it – trying to style and shape wet hair is just a waste
of time and effort.

Be careful when you dry your hair upside-down –
it can rough up the cuticle which leaves the hair
looking dull. Only do it occasionally if you want
to build up huge volume.

When using waxes and serums, the secret is
to start off with a tiny amount and add more
gradually if it is needed.

Always use a clean hairbrush – not one that is
clogged up with hair and product. You should
wash your brushes once a week in a little
shampoo and warm water.

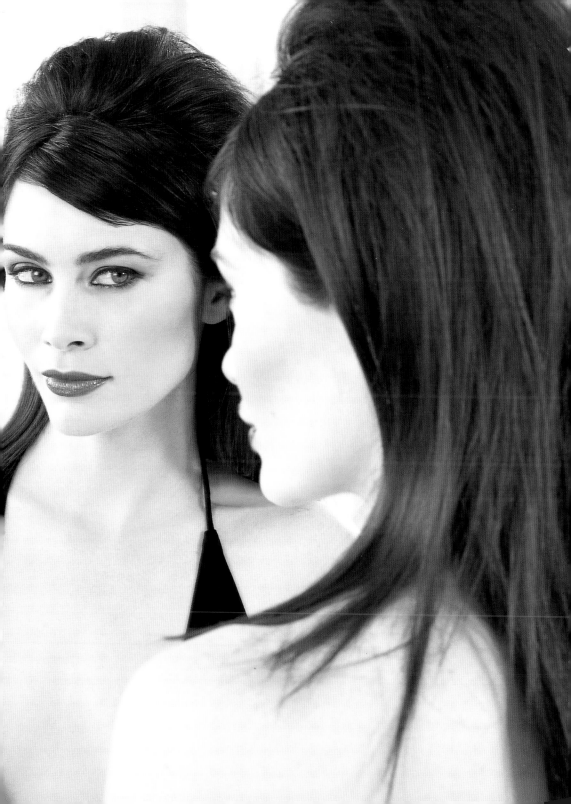

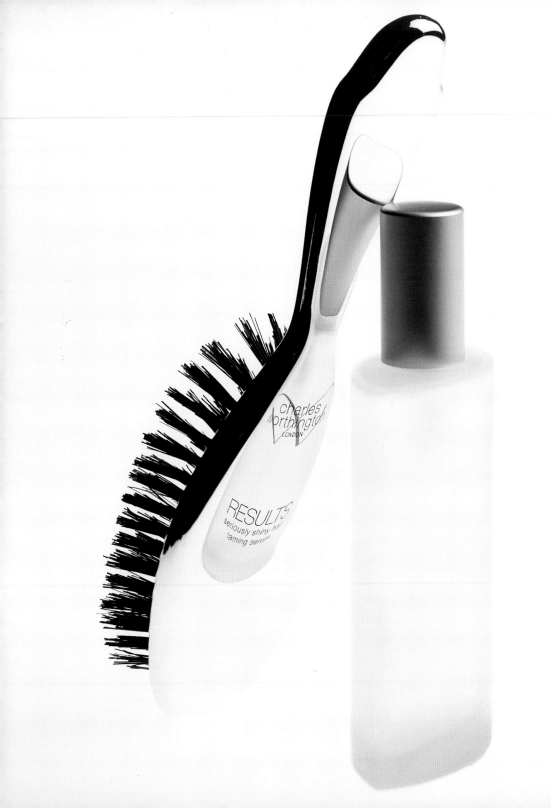

charles
Worthington
LONDON

RESULTS
seriously shiny hair
taming serum

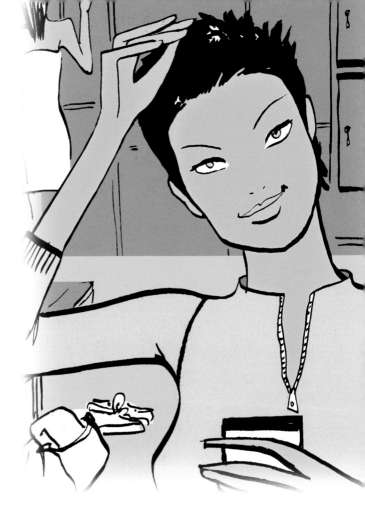

'It must be the effect** of living with looks-obsessed Chrissie and Jaz,' thinks Laura as she towel-dries her hair at the gym and contemplates making her gamine crop ... well, a little more interesting. Laura normally relishes the fact that she can jump out of the shower, blast her short hair dry and pull on her combats and trainers – all within ten minutes of finishing her kick-boxing class. Tonight, however, she has half an hour to kill before setting off for an

... laura glams up her gamine crop

important work party. 'Well, I might as well give it a go,' thinks Laura as she reaches into her gym bag for the little pot of styling wax that Chrissie gave her the night before. 'It'll gutsy-up your hair,' Chrissie had said – whatever that meant. Laura usually has little time

for Chrissie and her unsolicited beauty tips, but she wants to make an effort tonight. She works the wax into the ends as Chrissie had instructed, then blasts them dry, using her fingertips for lift. By the time she's finished, her hair looks sexy and tousled – as though

she's just climbed out of bed. Laura's impressed (in a rather understated, Laura kind of way). John, the devastatingly attractive assistant producer from Current Affairs, is likely to be at the party – and Laura's more than ready for a spot of networking – if that's what you want to call it.

colour me beautiful

Adding a touch of colour, whether it is permanent, semi-permanent or temporary, is a great way to perk up hair that is looking dull and lifeless, and a brilliant way to change your look or revolutionize your style. If the words 'shrinking' and 'violet' could never be used in the same sentence to describe you, then try adding a shock of bright colour – this adds punch to any hairstyle. The more faint-hearted can either boost and enhance their natural hair colour or get a little adventurous with some creative colour. How about a few strands of a contrasting shade around your face, for example? Or, what about getting just the very tips of your hair dipped in a daring bright colour? Either way, don't be afraid of colour; it can be really fun and opens up loads of opportunities for transforming yourself – à la Madonna, the mistress of reinvention.

something for the weekend?

The great thing about temporary colour is that it's, well ... temporary. It provides the perfect opportunity for trying out something new or for making an impact without causing any long-lasting and irreversible consequences. There'll be no crying over spilt milk with temporary colour!

It is always a good idea to pick your hairdresser's brains about colour before you launch yourself into the rainbow of choices and techniques available. Find out what colours they think will suit your skin tone and what formulations and techniques will have the best effect and results on your hair type.

colour wash

This easy wash-in, wash-out colour rinse lasts for just one shampoo and is good for subtle shade enhancement. Colour washes are also known as vegetable colours and are excellent for refreshing faded colour and conditioning the hair.

semi-permanent colour rinse

This is a vegetable-based dye that lasts for up to approximately 12 shampoos. You can only go darker or warmer than your natural colour.

coloured spray

As well as adding oomph to simpler styles, like plaits, this can be used to create an all-over effect. You could, for example, spray hair in a mist of silver to match a silver party dress – Barbarella, eat your heart out!

colour mousse

This is good for toning down brassiness or changing your colour for the night. It is best to seek professional advice as some leave a coloured 'cast' on the hair.

wax and pomade

These are applied after the hair has been dried and styled. It's always advisable to do a test strand with stronger colours to make sure it doesn't stain the hair and will wash out – especially if you have blonde or bleached hair. This product is best used on small areas.

hair mascara

The wand makes it really easy to streak colour through your hair. Use it around the front section of your hair and on the strands framing your face for best results. Be warned: test out hair mascaras at the beauty counter first as a colour that looks pretty in a tube can look pretty dull (or unnoticeable) on your hair.

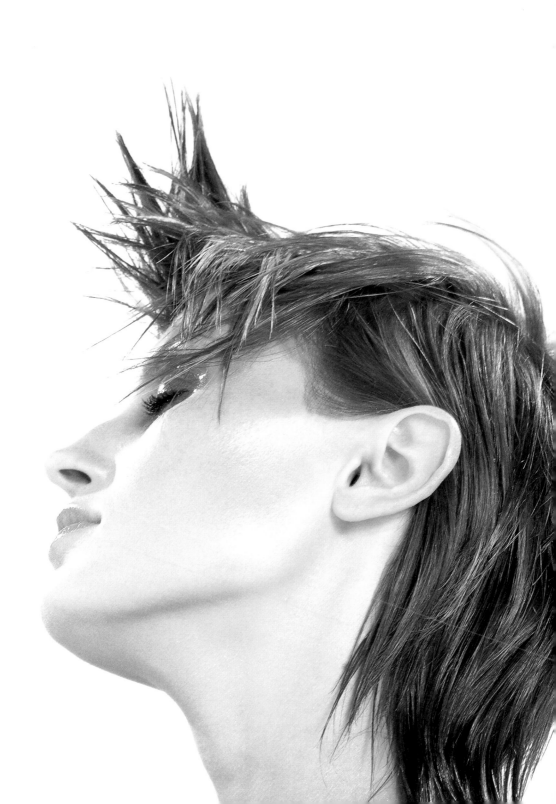

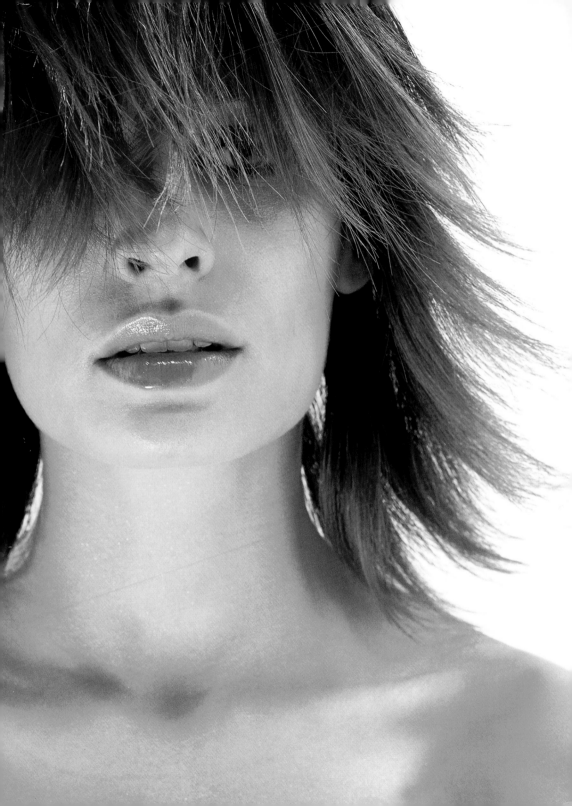

creative colour

Creative colour, as it's known in the salon, tends to be semi-permanent or permanent, so it's a great choice if you're feeling funky and want a look that's going to last longer than a couple of washes. As its name suggests, creative colour is where a hairstylist gets creative and even more artistic – your hair is a canvas on which colour application and technique converge. Some creative-colour techniques can produce quite radical results, so talk it through with your hairdresser and make sure you know exactly what you're letting yourself in for. Your gorgeous tie-dye locks may not be appreciated if you work in a bank or law firm!

If you're longing to try techniques like dip-dyeing or tie-dyeing but think they sound a bit radical and long-lasting, you can cheat by colouring hairpieces and then weaving them into your hair.

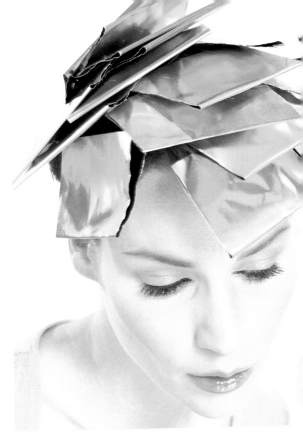

dip-dyeing

This technique (left), inspired by the art of dip-dyeing clothes, is where just the very ends of your hair are coloured. It works best on natural, mid-length to long hair and you can use either subtle or vibrant colours. For the most dramatic results, have your ends dip-dyed in a contrasting colour to your natural shade. For example, if your hair is dark brown or black, dip-dye the ends pillar-box red.

couture colour

Your hair is shaded with colour to personalize and complement your haircut, making it unique to you. This type of colour enhances movement and emphasizes a dramatic line.

tonal blast

This is a more subtle version of dip-dyeing that works best on short to mid-length textured haircuts. The ends of the hair are coloured and then a semi-permanent colour wash is applied over the top to give extra brightness and a strong tone of colour. A tonal blast can be done on all natural or coloured hair, with the exception of hair that has been dyed black.

3-D lights

Slices of hair are coloured with shades of blonde all over the head; darker blonde is applied at the roots and lighter blonde to the ends to give a sun-kissed look. This works best on short to mid-length hair and can be done on all shades of natural or coloured blonde hair.

hidden colour

Sections of hair are taken from underneath and coloured, which makes 'work-to-play' hair easy – clip up your hair to reveal the drama below. This works best on all natural hair colours and on mid-length to long hair.

duo colour

The hair is either coloured lighter on top and darker underneath or darker on top and lighter underneath. This can be done on all natural or coloured hair and works best on mid-length to long hair. Trio colour involves using three contrasting colours.

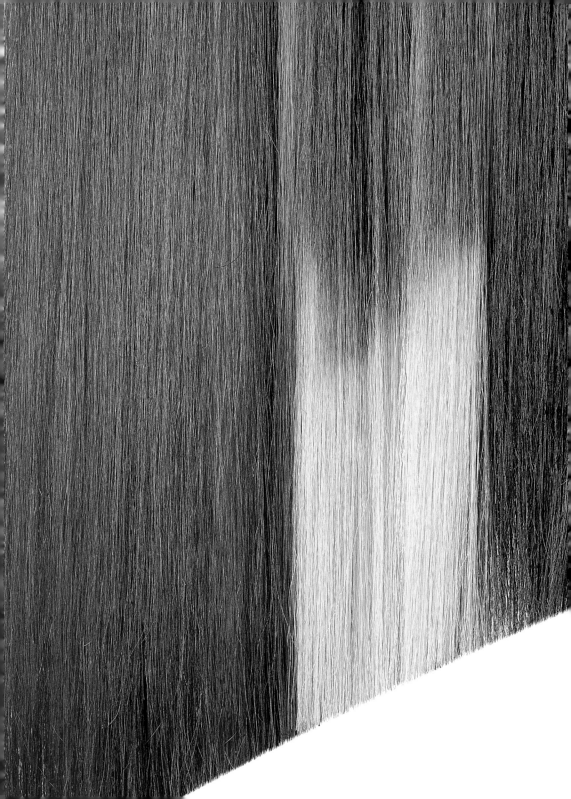

hang loose

spoiling themselves at the spa

Wrapped in fluffy white robes, the girls sat clutching cups of calming herbal tea while having their toes pedicured in the calm cream reception area of their favourite spa. Their faces were as long as Chrissie's newly-painted acrylic nails. It had not been a good week, so they had decided to cheer themselves up with a little bit of pampering. Good old Polly had even offered to pay for Jaz, who could not have afforded to go otherwise. The soothing tinkle of the feng-shui water wall and the prospect of a massage with hot stones (the latest beauty treatment) had already helped to lift their spirits.

'Poor Jaz,' thought Polly. Her dream work placement on *Gloss* magazine had not turned out to be quite as glamorous as she had expected. For the past week she had been incarcerated in the windowless fashion cupboard, sorting out the tights and set free only to fetch organic wheatgrass juice for Imogen, the fashion editor. As for meeting a fashion designer, she was about as likely to meet Elvis.

'Pass me that copy of *The Rainbow*, please Jaz. I need to work on my new image,' barked Chrissie. She had become even more obsessed with her looks since Pout had proclaimed her 'too womanly' to join their band. She was devastated about it but, in true Chrissie style, only for about two seconds. Instead, she had accepted the job of receptionist at Devastation Records that Steve had offered her by way of compensation. He had hinted that if she took the job, there was a chance that she might be 'discovered'. 'Too right I will,' Chrissie had thought, resolving there and then to be the most glamorous (and girliest) receptionist ever. 'And to think I wore my lucky red dress,' she thought aloud to herself, while admiring her newly-painted, mink-coloured toenails (the perfect accompaniment to her long, honey-coloured calves, she thought).
'Yes, but look at what you wore with the red dress,'

pointed out Laura, characteristically as blunt as the cut of her boyish crop. 'Those turquoise tights that Jaz persuaded you to wear looked ridiculous!'

'Laura, don't be mean to Chrissie,' said Polly, looking up from the work file she had brought along with her for light reading – anything to take her mind off the fact that Simon had not called. Worse still, his once-flirtatious e-mails had become very brisk and matter-of-fact. And to top it all, Polly was feeling really guilty about Harry, who seemed to have finally woken up to her existence. He had actually paid her a compliment about her new 'messy' hair (as he called it) and had even presented her with a bunch of flowers – even though they were carnations.

'I think I might go for the slimming seaweed wrap,' declared Kate, who had been scanning the menu of beauty treatments. Out of all the girls, Kate secretly had something to celebrate. She had managed to lose a bit of weight since switching to a new, low-fat brand of biscuit that was being trial-tested at Crunch. Matthew was currently racking his brains, trying to think of a name for them. Kate, however, had already thought of one. It was time to convince her gorgeous boss that her talents stretched to more than just typing letters and doing the filing.

Laura was also studying the treatments on offer. Beauty spas were not usually her thing, but she'd willingly agreed when Polly'd suggested it. She had to do something to get John's attention. At the TV party where she had planned to 'bump' into him, he had spent the entire time talking to a girl with long, curly hair who was wearing a flowery frock. 'Chrissie's worried about looking too womanly, but maybe my problem,' thought Laura, as she helped herself to an apple, 'is that I'm not womanly enough.' Still, it was never too late for a cynical 26-year-old TV researcher to learn a beauty trick or two.

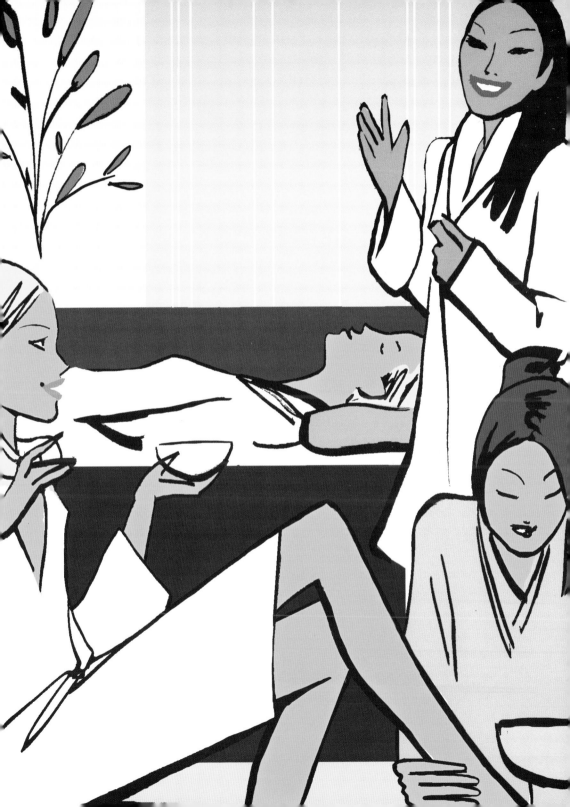

straight talking

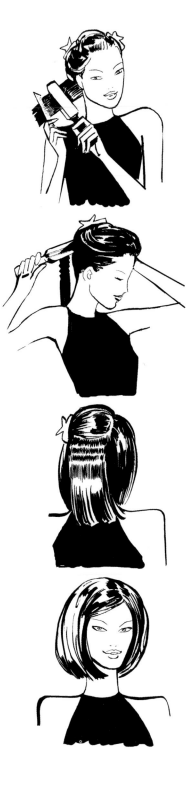

Straight is not as straightforward as you might think. You can take your pick from straight and dishevelled, straight and sleek or straight with lots of volume. There are as many ways to wear your hair loose as there are shades of lipstick. Hair worn down is a great seduction tool: you can indulge in lots of flirtatious ploys, like tossing it back or playfully running your fingers through it (although strictly speaking, this is a no-no as it can make hair look greasy).That said, the secret to great date hair is a style that somebody else wants to run their fingers through ...

big straight hair

Big straight hair is all about boosting thickness without weighing down the hair. Here's the lowdown:

you need
Wide flat brush (ideally a paddle brush) • hairdryer • crimping irons • straightening irons • sectioning clips • non-aerosol hairspray

1 Follow the instructions on page 18 for blow-drying and straightening your hair with straightening irons.

2 Pin the top layers of your hair out of the way, using the sectioning clips.

3 Take the underneath layers, section by section, and lightly spritz the root area with hairspray to protect it from the heat of the crimping iron, then crimp the hair close to the roots.

4 When you have crimped the roots of all the underneath layers, gently comb the crimped sections out and then let the hair you have pinned away fall over the top.

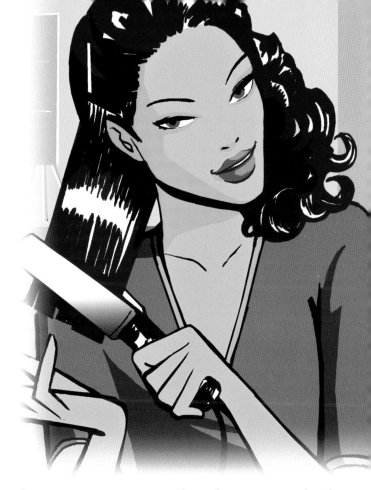

Spurred on by her weight loss (it was a good start) and her indulgent day at the spa (she definitely felt more toned after the seaweed wrap), Kate decides that Sunday night is going to be

... kate takes her power bob straight

'an achieve salon-style hair at home' night. She furtively eyes the carrier bag that contains her latest purchase. It's over a month since she walked into her hairdresser's and demanded a power bob. What she had been given – a shoulder-length bob-shaped cut – was as close to a power bob as you can get when you possess flowing, unruly titian locks. But Kate hankers after bone-straight hair – the mark of the sleek, sophisticated

career babe. She is positive that with the right hair she could get ahead in the Crunch marketing department. Like a woman with a serious mission, she plugs in her new straightening irons to let them heat up while she sections off her hair as instructed by the accompanying booklet. She can hardly believe the transformation that takes place as she carefully runs the irons down each section. In less than half an hour she goes from

pre-Raphaelite maiden to a smart, take-me-seriously hotshot. She knows that she can't do this sort of thing too often (overuse of straightening irons being very damaging to the hair), but once in a while can't possibly hurt. Delighted with her new image (she even looks as sharp and business-like as Polly), she decides that tomorrow is the day to broach the subject of accompanying Matthew on that important conference.

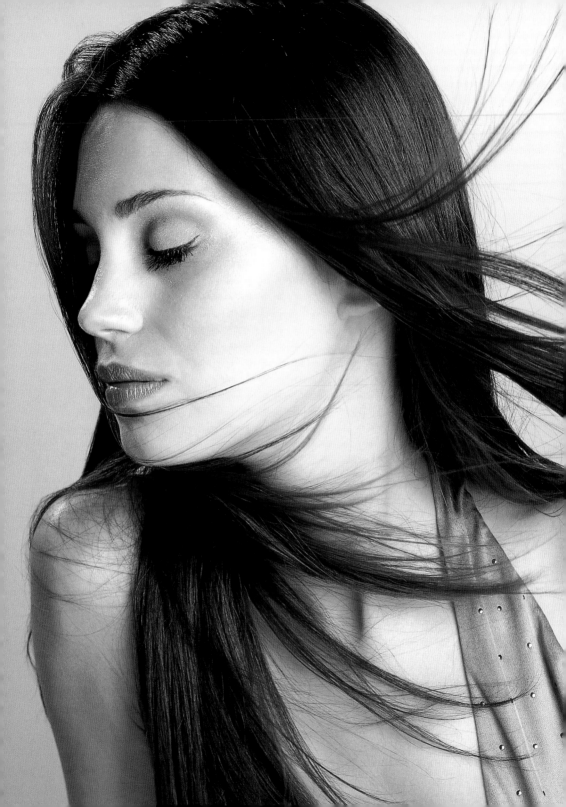

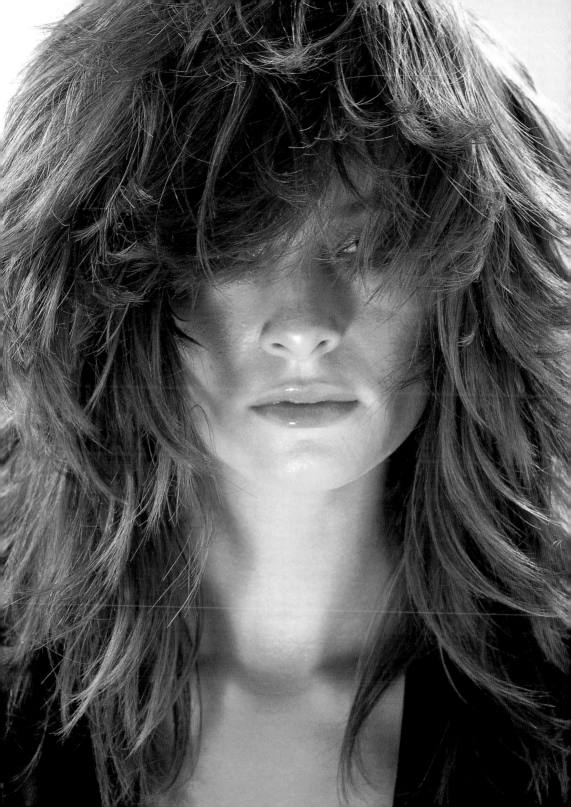

blades

There's straight, there's big straight and then there's 'Gucci-style' straight, which leaves your hair looking like blades of grass all over. (Hence the salon-speak for this look is simply 'blades'.) It's a very sharp look that makes your hair seem almost crispy. But be warned: this technique involves hot straightening irons and is potentially dehydrating to the hair if used regularly, so it is best saved for big dates only.

you need
hairdryer • straightening brush • pump-action hairspray • straightening irons

1 Follow the instructions on page 18 for blow-drying your hair straight.

2 Using a pump-action rather than an aerosol hairspray, spritz the hair until it is quite damp. (A pump-action hairspray releases a higher volume of product, which makes the hair damper.) Do this evenly down the entire length of your hair.

3 Take a small 2.5-cm (1-inch) wide section of hair and slowly run the straightening irons down it, from the roots to the ends.

4 Repeat this process all over the head, being sure to straighten the underneath layers and not just the top section. This should leave the hair totally separated into small individual 'blades'.

bed-head hair

There is something very sexy about slightly dishevelled or shaggy hair, also known as 'bed-head hair' because it looks like you've just climbed out of bed and not bothered to brush it. On long hair, this look is also labelled 'Rock Chick' – messy, but sexy, as sported by Chrissie Hynde, Courtney Love and Marianne Faithful.

you need
Light-hold mousse or gel spray • hairdryer • paddle brush • hairspray

1 Apply a little mousse or gel spray to the root area of the hair using your fingers to work it through.

2 Rough-dry the hair. Instead of sectioning off the hair and blow-drying each piece separately, randomly blast the hair with the hairdryer, gently roughing it up with your fingers. This will maximize the volume and give a really shaggy finish.

3 Lightly spritz with hairspray to hold the look.

short and spiky

Don't think that just because you've got short hair, you have limited styling options. There's a lot you can do with short hair – you can make it soft, sexy and tousled; slick it back neatly for understated glossy elegance; decorate it with pretty hair slides and grips; or spike it up for a groovy, street-chick look – all you need is a range of good styling products, some basic tools and a little bit of know-how. This funky textured look (right) is a great way to make short hair more gutsy, and will certainly get you noticed.

you need
Strong-hold gel • hairdryer and diffuser • hairspray

1 Apply a generous amount of strong-hold gel to wet hair, using your fingers to distribute the product evenly through to the ends. Gently work the hair into spikes, spacing them evenly over the head.

2 Dry your hair with your head tipped over, using a diffuser to help keep all of the spikes intact.

3 Finally, spray your hair with hairspray to add extra hold and shine.

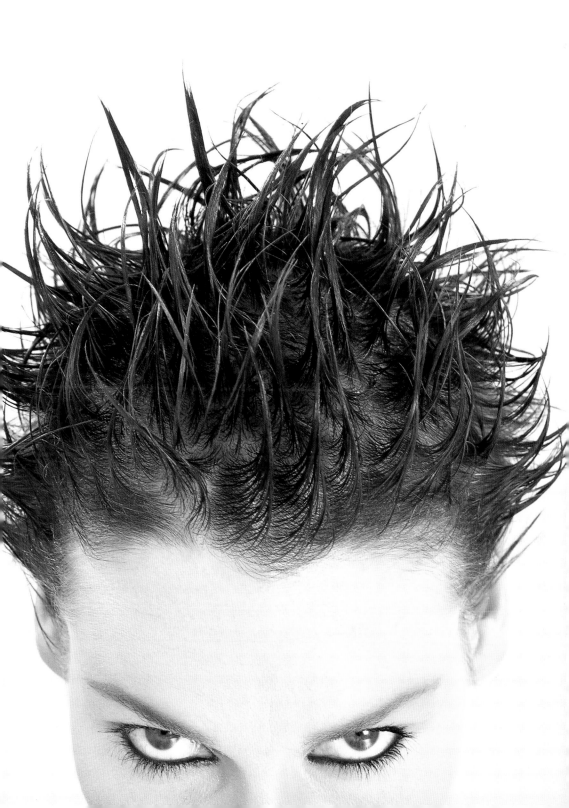

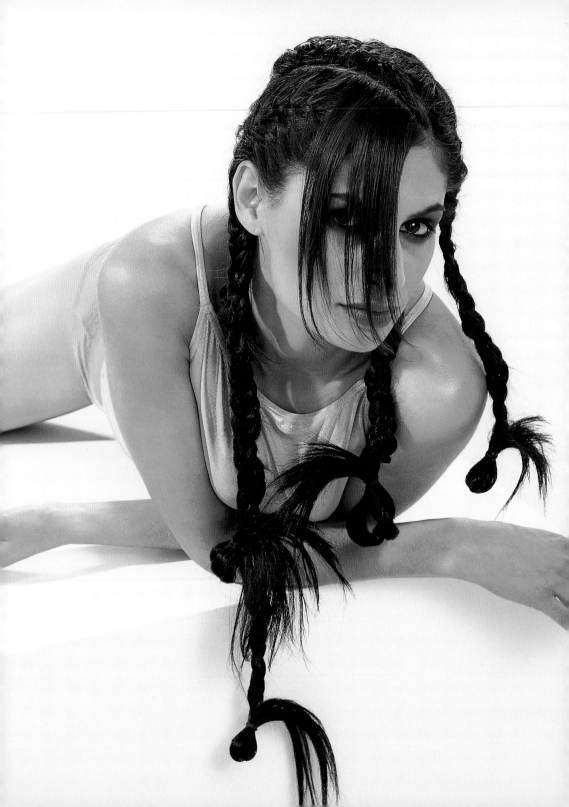

plait it, braid it

Plaits are not just for schoolgirls – they can look very elegant, very hip or very sexy. There are loads of variations – from a single braid hanging straight down your back to a whole headful of braiding finished with beads. If you don't want all of your hair in a plait, just braid a small section of the hair anywhere you like to add extra texture and interest. The most popular way to do this is to plait a small section on either side of the face and then take these around the side of the head and clip them at the back. Very Guinevere!

the multiplait

This is a very beautiful, very simple style of wearing your hair down your back in a neat, elegant, textural plait.

you need
Comb • sectioning clips • three covered elastic bands • hairspray or anti-frizz serum

HAIR SNIP

TO AVOID HAVING A BIG CHUNKY BAND AT THE END OF YOUR PLAIT, FINISH IT OFF BY LIGHTLY BACKCOMBING THE TIPS OF THE HAIR. ALTERNATIVELY, USE CLEAR, SNAG-FREE ELASTIC BANDS FOR LARGER PLAITS OR BEADS FOR SMALLER PLAITS.

FRENCH PLAITS LOOK NEATER AND STAY TIGHTER FOR LONGER IF YOU ADD IN VERY SMALL SECTIONS OF HAIR AT EACH TURN. ALWAYS PLAIT THEM TIGHT AGAINST THE SCALP.

FOR A PLAIT WITH A DIFFERENCE, WEAVE IN COLOURFUL RIBBONS OR STRIPS OF LEATHER. YOU CAN ALSO DECORATE PLAITS WITH FLOWERS AND FEATHERS.

1 Divide your hair into three sections: one on the left, one at the back and one on the right.

2 Divide the left section into three, plait it near the nape and secure it with a hair band.

3 Plait the right section in the same way, leaving the middle section unplaited.

4 Then plait all three sections together for an interesting combination of textures.

5 Finally, use hairspray or an anti-frizz serum to flatten any stray hairs.

sexy plaits

These are sexy, bad-girl plaits!

you need
Comb • sectioning clips • three snag-free elastic bands • shine spray • straightening irons

1 Divide the hair into three sections from the front of the head to the nape, leaving out a small section at the front to flop seductively over one eye.

2 French-plait the first section tightly onto the scalp, following the shape of the head. This is important as it will ensure that the plait is tight towards the nape.

3 Leave about 15 cm (6 in) unplaited at the end. Fold this back and secure it with a snag-free elastic.

4 Repeat with the other two plaits, then spritz the hair with shine spray (see opposite).

5 Finish by straightening the loose front section.

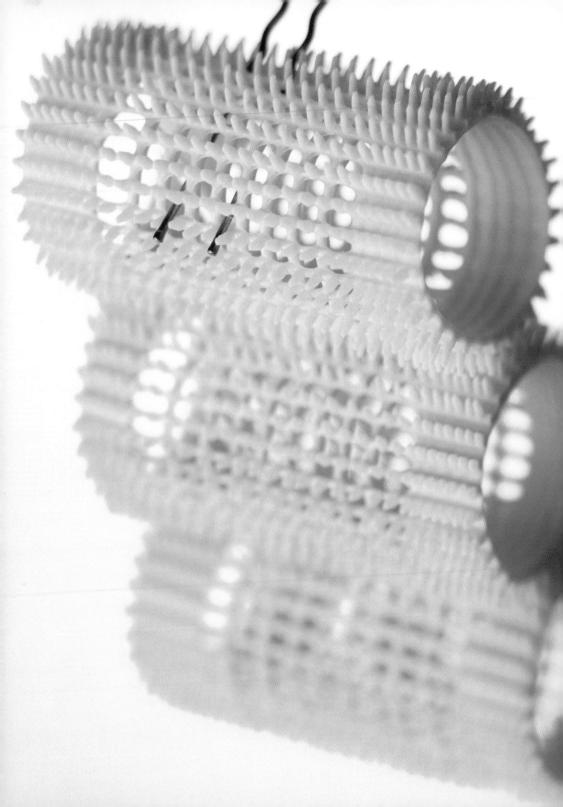

girls with curls

In the same way as girls with the most beautiful curly locks at times lust after flat-ironed hair, those born with naturally straight tresses long for a cascade of tumbling curls. Maybe it's because the grass is always greener ... Straightening or curling, you can't defy nature permanently, but you can have a lot of fun.

Curls come in many different guises: from the softest Madonna-style wave to tight corkscrews and romantic Jane Austen ringlets. Even if your hair is naturally as straight as a ruler, it's easy to create the curls of your dreams at home.

wavy hair

The best way to achieve long-lasting, glossy curls is to use curling tongs. It is important to work on freshly washed hair (too much product on the hair will make it look dull when you use tongs).

you need

Comb • hairspray • curling tongs • glossing spray

1 Starting at the nape of the neck, divide the hair into quite chunky sections (about 9 cm/3.5 in wide).

2 Lightly spray the first section with hairspray to ensure a longer-lasting curl.

3 Comb it through to remove any product build-up before clamping the tongs over the ends of the section, making sure they are completely tucked in.

4 Gently wind the tongs up, making sure that all the hair is covering the metal barrel. Hold for about 4–10 seconds, depending on the heat of the tongs and the curl required, then gently unwind. (Be careful not to run your fingers through the curled section.)

5 Repeat this process until all of your hair has been tonged, then lightly spray it with a light glossing spray to finish.

ringlets

If you have naturally curly hair, creating ringlets is easy. This technique is also a good way to avoid frizzy curls.

you need

Serum • styling gel • comb • finishing spray

1 Simply rub serum and gel together in the palm of one hand. Apply to wet hair and comb it through.

2 Leave your hair to dry naturally and the hair will form ringlets. For a bit of extra help, take sections of hair and twist them around your finger before leaving to dry.

3 For a glossy finish, lightly spritz with finishing spray.

If you have straight hair, there are several methods of creating ringlets. The old-fashioned technique of 'ragging', using torn-up bits of cloth (strips of J-cloth works especially well), has made a twenty-first century comeback. Once mastered, it is quicker and better than using rollers.

you need

Medium-hold styling spray • strips of cloth • hairdryer and diffuser (optional)

1 Start by spritzing the hair with medium-hold styling spray (use quite a lot to give a firm, springy curl).

2 Beginning at the nape of the neck, divide the hair into sections depending on the size of ringlet required. (Continued on page 44.)

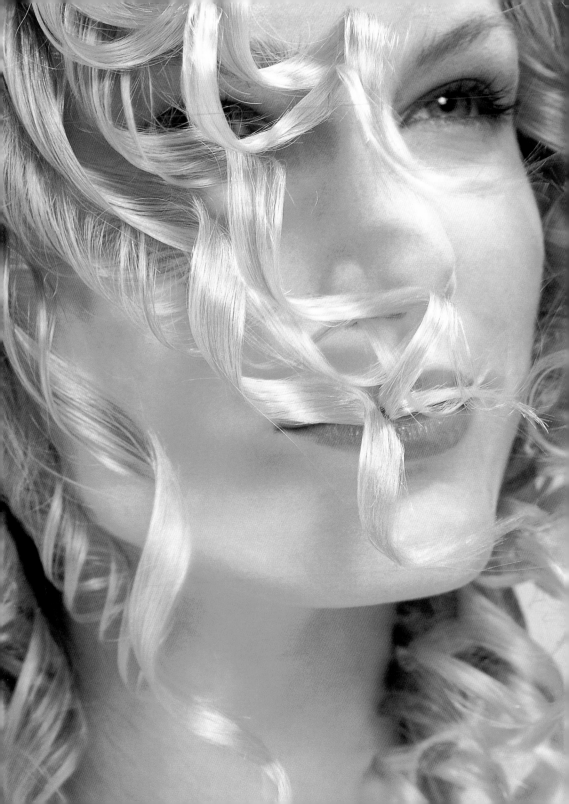

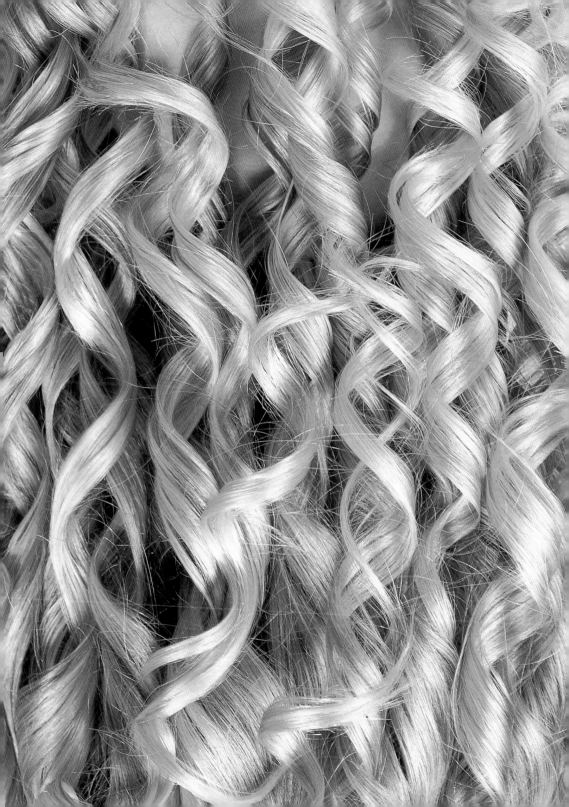

3 Wrap the hair around the cloth, being careful to tuck in the ends neatly. For a more defined ringlet, slightly twist each section as you wind it up.

4 Once the hair is wound tightly around the strip of cloth, snug to the scalp, tie the two ends of the cloth together.

5 When all the hair is tied, either leave it to dry naturally (the rags are comfortable enough to sleep in), or use a hairdryer and diffuser – but this can be time-consuming.

6 When you are sure that the hair is dry, start to remove the rags, beginning at the nape of the neck.

7 When all the rags have been removed, use your fingers to gently break up the curls, depending on how curly or defined you want the final effect.

afro-style

You don't even need to have curly hair to create a cloud of tight Afro curls. Even poker-straight tresses can be transformed to get this effect.

you need
Strong setting lotion • strips of silver foil • wide-tooth comb

1 Spritz the hair thoroughly with strong setting lotion to give a more defined curl.

2 Follow the instructions for ragging (see above), but take much smaller sections of hair and instead of winding the hair around strips of cloth, use small pieces of foil.

3 When you remove the pieces of foil, instead of running your fingers through the hair, use a wide-tooth comb. This will totally separate the curls, leaving you with a perfect Afro.

big curls

If you're not satisfied with Madonna-style waves or a headful of ringlets, then big curls (with a capital B) are the order of the day. Reach out for the hot rollers for a bit of va-va voom.

you need
Mousse • hairdryer • hairspray • heated rollers

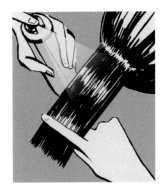

1 To create the perfect foundation for a hot-roller set, apply mousse to the root area of freshly washed hair. Then, using the warm setting on your hairdryer, dry the mousse into the hair.

2 Take a section of hair, making sure it's not wider than the actual roller, and spray it evenly with hairspray.

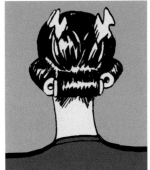

3 Wind the section around the end of the first roller, tucking in the ends. Make sure that the roller sits firmly against the scalp as this will create root lift and a much bouncier curl.

4 When you've finished putting all of the hair in rollers, apply a coat of hairspray evenly all over. Leave the rollers in for about 10 minutes before gently unrolling them. Don't tug or pull the rollers out.

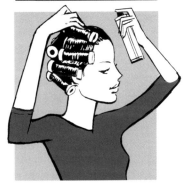

HAIR SNIP

MAKE SURE THAT THE ENDS OF THE HAIR ARE TUCKED IN WHEN YOU CURL THE HAIR AROUND THE ROLLERS, TONGS OR RAGS, OTHERWISE YOU WILL END UP WITH A FISH-HOOK EFFECT AT THE END OF THE CURL.

WAIT FOR THE HOT ROLLERS TO GO COLD BEFORE REMOVING THEM AS THIS WILL CLOSE THE CUTICLES OF THE HAIR AND SET THE CURLS.

SPRAY EACH SECTION WITH SHINE SPRAY AS YOU REMOVE THE ROLLER TO GUARANTEE GLOSSY AND VOLUMINOUS CURLS.

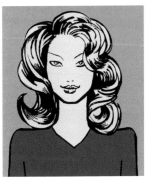

Jaz is dreading the prospect of another boring afternoon in the fashion cupboard, bagging up clothes from the glamorous shoots that she never gets to go on. Imogen announces that she's simply going have to go home with another one of her stress headaches (although Jaz can't see exactly what stress her boss is under since all she does is chat on the phone all day to her friends, dahling). She wonders, would Jaz mind going to the launch of Blast, Jean-Paul's new perfume, after work in her place? Jaz would just about manage ... Stifling a squeal, she tries to look nonchalant, but not very effectively. Anyway, the coast is now clear for the rest of the afternoon and she has a party to get ready for. Jaz has been dying to try on that amazing purple dress from Coletta, and perhaps a new hairstyle would be just the thing to cheer her up. Emboldened, she manages to get herself an appointment with *Gloss*'s favoured hairstylist, Adam, and begs him to create something awesome for the launch that

... jaz goes crazy with the crimpers

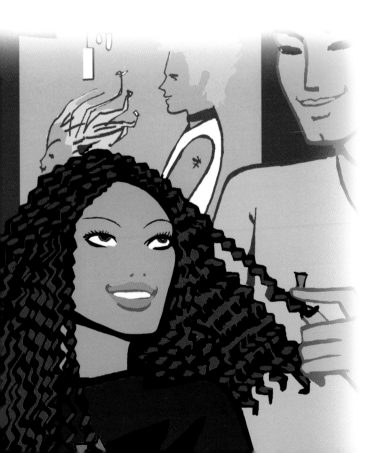

night. He patiently crimps every bit of her long, dark glossy hair, backcombing it at the roots for extra volume. 'Hmm, not bad,' thinks Jaz. Flicking through a back issue of *Gloss*, she spots a picture of a catwalk model with plaits wrapped around the side of her head. Adam obligingly braids the front sections of her hair into four small plaits, tying the ends with coloured ribbon. The effect is Kate Bush meets Guinevere – altogether quite pleasing. Jaz is thrilled. Falling off her precarious pin stiletto heels, she rushes out of the salon towards her oh-so-chic destination, but not before giving Adam a massive hug in gratitude. 'I'll do you a favour,' she shrieks, almost tripping up as she tries to hail a cab. 'I won't hold my breath,' thinks Adam, 'but she is a real cutie.'

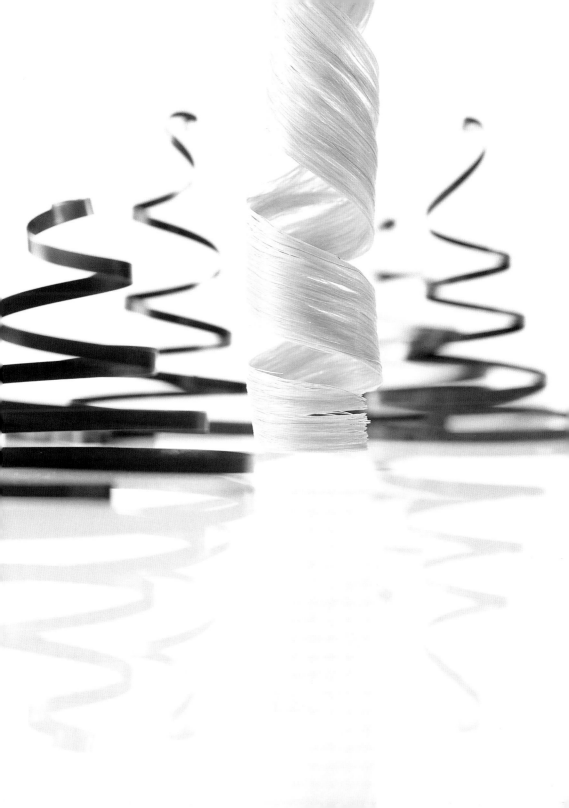

glamourtime tips

1 Accessorize, accessorize, accessorize. There are so many clever, simple accessories on the market that can be used to make an instant change from dawn to night.

2 Glam up any style by using a sparkle gel or spray glitter along your parting.

3 If you are going to a hot, sweaty party, backcomb the hair at the root to keep the hair big all night.

4 Outshine any rivals: to polish the hair and make it super-shiny, rub a few drops of serum into the palm of your hand, then sweep a large make-up brush across your hand and smooth it down the hair shaft. This is especially effective on long hair.

5 Apply coloured hair mascara – in gold, copper, blonde or a shade lighter than your own – to strands around your face for instant do-it-yourself highlights.

6 Scent your hair by spraying a cloud of perfume into the air and then walking through it. Hair holds perfume really well, so this seductive little trick should create wafts of gorgeousness every time you flick your hair or turn your head.

7 Hold your hair away from your face with beautiful jewelled clips, or pin it back with a big fake flower.

8 For a super-quick, super-dramatic solution, use a ponytail extension (see page 70).

9 Gently curl the ends of ruler-straight hair using tongs to create contrasting texture.

10 Randomly crimp sections of your hair to create volume and a multitextured look.

11 Twist curly sections into full bundles and secure them with glitzy hair grips.

12 Jazz up poker-straight hair by randomly plaiting sections throughout, even plaiting coloured ribbon into them.

13 If you're working the party circuit and styling your hair a lot, you may find that your hair becomes heavy and lank due to a build-up of products. Simply use a detoxifying shampoo for a thorough cleanse.

14 Experiment with a wig – why not be someone else for a night?

15 Overuse of heated styling appliances can damage or dry the hair, so always make sure that you follow instructions carefully. If you are concerned that your hair is becoming dry, then use a rich, conditioning hair treatment or mask once a week to replenish moisture levels.

16 To give your naturally straight hair a bit of texture, plait damp hair before you go to bed. When you wake up, apply a little serum to your fingertips and run them through the hair to undo the plaits. Or, for a quick fix, apply hairspray to dry hair and plait it. Leave it for half an hour and then undo the plaits to get crinkly waves.

17 When choosing your parting, look at what you're wearing. Pick out a feature like the shape of your neckline and follow this when styling your parting.

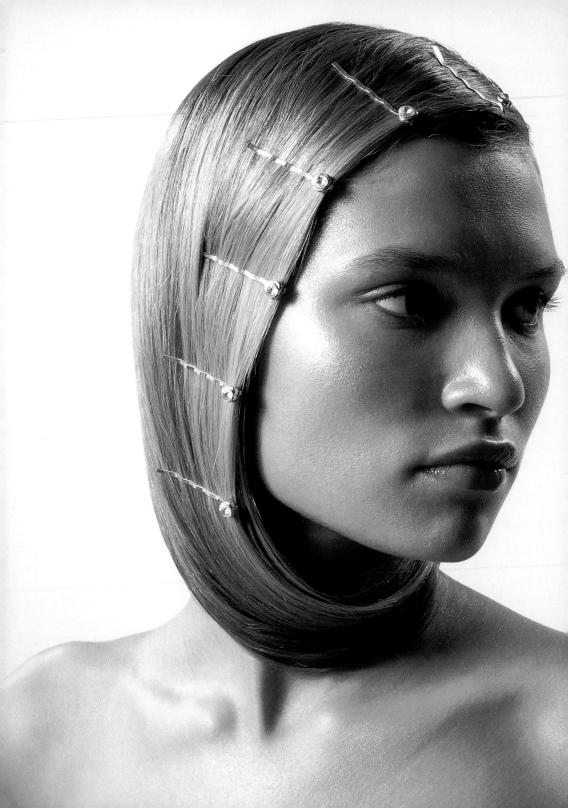

hair dressing

Hair accessories, like fringes (bangs), are a very personal thing. Some might love a big fake lily poking out from behind the ear; others may not. Hair slides, clips, feathers, flowers and all sorts of glittery bits and bobs can make a great finishing flourish, but they go in and out of fashion faster than you can say 'Kirby grip', so don't waste money on expensive pieces, and be sure to play around with them first before buying them.

tiaras and headbands

Tiaras can look great with long or short hair, but the trick is to wear them with irony (think Courtney Love rather than royalty). We can thank fashion gurus for the revival of headscarves and bandanas. A brightly patterned scarf worn bandana-style over long, straight hair can look very cool. (It's also a great way to cover up on a bad-hair day!)

Head bands come in a range of widths, materials and finishes, whether you want to opt for a minimal strip of leather or a kitsch band with beaded flowers attached to the side. Make sure they fit properly and comfortably.

do-it-yourself accessories

It's amazing what you can make in the way of hair accessories using old pieces of jewellery. You can wire brooches onto combs; glue beads or sequins onto slides; or thread beads onto wire and attach them to hair grips. You can even use a diamanté necklace or bracelet to decorate your hair – simply drape it over your hair and secure it in place with a few matt hair grips.

Glue decorative coloured feathers onto thin strips of leather – either natural or dyed a bright colour – and then attach them to matt hair grips.

Wrap fine florist's wire around the stems of fresh flowers, individually or arranged in small posies, and attach them to hair slides, grips or combs.

clips

Beautiful glittery, jewelled, beaded or feathered clips are one of the best and easiest forms of hair ornament. They can either be attached randomly throughout the hair or placed at the side to keep hair back from the face.

flowers

A big flower – real or fake – pinned behind the ear or at the back of the head is a great way to 'dress up' not only your hair, but also a simple outfit for a big date.

glitter sprays and gels

You only have to look at the big trend for iridescent and glittery face and body make-up to realize that sparkle and shine are definitely 'in'. Try adding a bit of glitter to strands of hair around the face to brighten up your complexion and put you in the party mood.

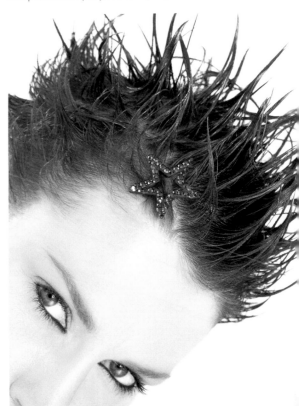

great lengths

If you want to hang loose but your hair doesn't even reach your jaw line, don't despair. You don't have to wait for your hair to grow, you can get a head start by faking it with hairpieces, extensions and wigs. No longer the domain of the follically challenged, these hairpieces are amazingly realistic, and, more to the point, they allow you to experiment with looks you could otherwise never achieve. Sport a sexy, gamine crop by day and a Rapunzel-like mane by night!

faking it

Clip-on extensions and hairpieces are a great way to add volume or length to your hair. But in order to weave some practical magic with a hairpiece, you do need to have a bit of length already, as they look better when they blend with existing hair (see page 70 for instructions on how to attach them).

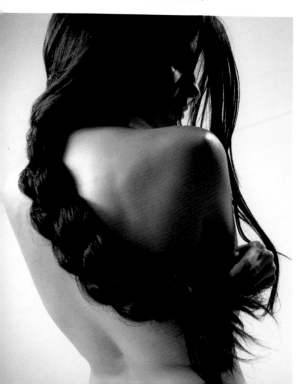

To achieve extreme long hair', attach five to ten narrow 60-cm (23½-in) hairpieces from the nape to the crown of the head using toupee clips. These are slightly rounded so they sit nice and flat on the head. If your hair is shorter, you could try fake ponytails or plaits, which are attached with clips or combs.

wig tips

1 To make a wig look more natural, have it cut on your head by your hairdresser (razor-cutting techniques tend to work and look best).

2 To give a wig extra body and to make it look less fake, try crimping the roots.

3 If you have a long, straight wig in a colour that is a close match to your own hair, a great trick is to cut small sections out of it and pull strands of your own hair through it. Blending the wig with your own hair in this way not only makes the wig look more convincing, but also prevents it from slipping off your head.

4 If you are wearing a wig over long hair and want it to sit more closely to the scalp, cover your head with the foot of a popsock and put the wig on over the top.

5 When washing wigs or hairpieces, always seek professional advice; not all wigs are made from human hair and they may need special care and attention.

6 Be very careful when you handle wigs and hairpieces – they are woven onto a weft so they are very delicate.

7 Ask to see the actual wig or hairpiece you wish to buy, as natural hairpieces are different in colour and may vary from the colour chart.

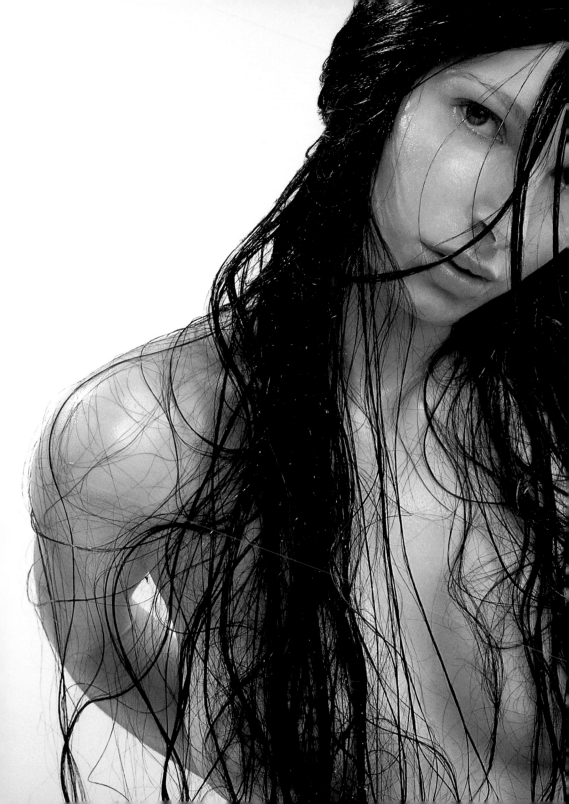

emergency quick fixes

1 To revive or add volume to hair when there is no time to wash it, simply spritz the roots with blow-drying spray and then dry the hair, focusing on the root area.

2 If your hair starts to droop, tip your head upside down and spritz the roots with hairspray. Don't be tempted to put too much product on the ends of the hair as it will just drag it down.

3 A handy trick: if your hair has collapsed from too much energetic dancing in a club, or if you don't have access to a blow-dryer, spritz the roots with hairspray and use the hand-dryer in the cloakroom to dry it.

4 When you are pinning up your hair with hair grips, lightly backcomb the roots as this will give a longer-lasting hold.

5 If all else fails, tie your hair back in a low ponytail, securing it at the nape. For an extra-tight hold, wrap it with a piece of wet string instead of a hair band – the string will contract as it dries.

SOS tool kit

Make space for the following in your bag and you need never have another bad-hair moment again!

comb or brush
This one goes without saying.

covered elastic band
With one of these you can always pull your hair back in an emergency.

multifunction styling spray
Use this for holding updos in place or giving an emergency lift to hair that's looking a little limp.

five matt hair grips
These will enable you to fix your hair in a sleek chignon or updo and go straight out from work to play. Matt hair grips don't slip out of the hair and don't show as much as shiny ones.

serum
This silicone-based wonder product will smooth out any frizz and give a sleek, shiny finish.

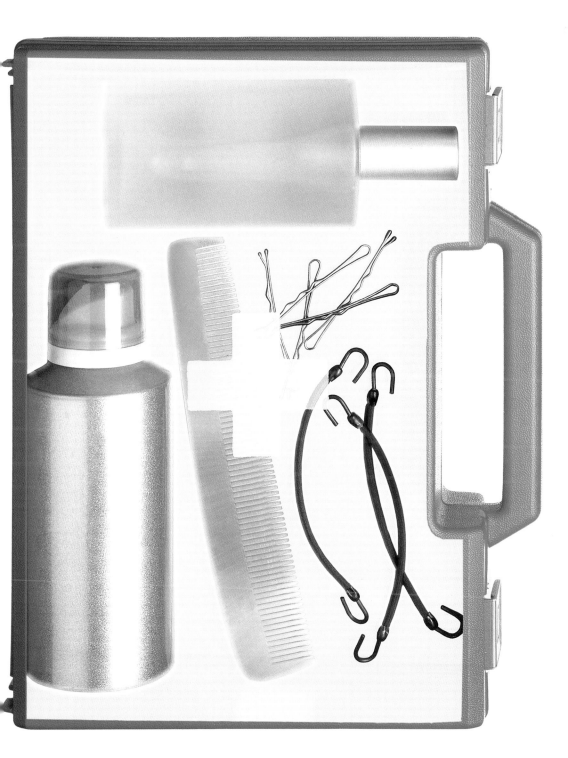

updos

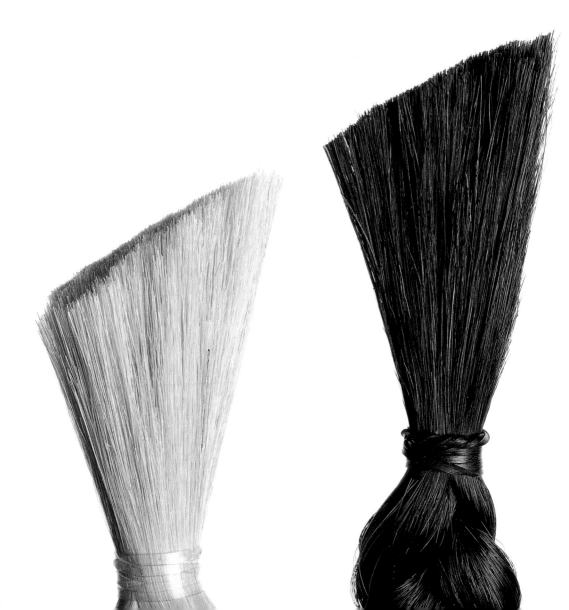

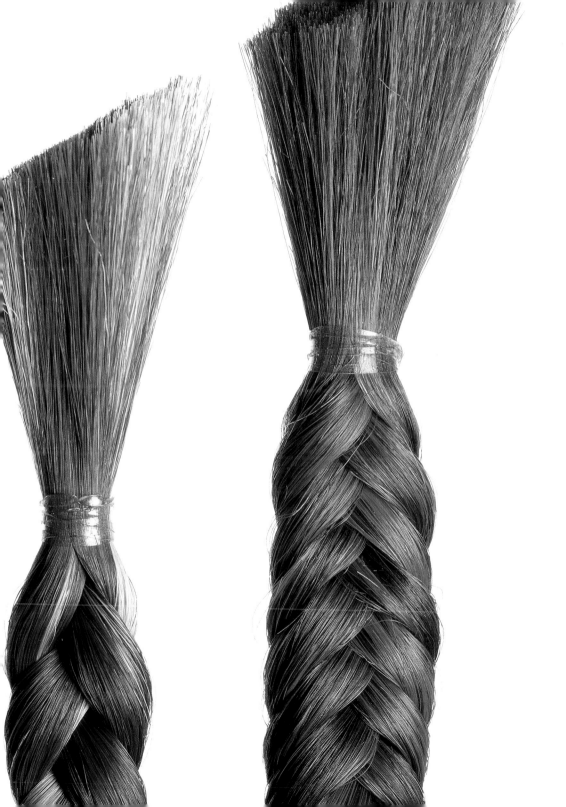

a quiet night in washing hair

'The pizzas have arrived,' yelled Polly, entering the kitchen with a stack of boxes. It was Thursday and the girls were having a quiet night in washing their hair. Things were looking up for all of them. Chrissie had finally cajoled Laura into going on that double date – drinks and dinner in the Rush bar tomorrow. Meanwhile, Kate's boss had asked her to attend the biscuit conference in Birmingham. This – she couldn't believe her luck – was to be followed by a gala dinner. 'OK, so it's not exactly a date,' she had told the girls, 'but I'm certainly not planning to talk to Matthew about custard creams all night!'

The girls plonked themselves down on the floor around Polly's chic, Balinese-style coffee table to eat their pizza. 'Oh God, I'm almost too tired to eat,' said Jaz, slumped on a cream beanbag, a vision in a beige-and-lime print shirtdress. She was permanently exhausted these days, ironing tights at *Gloss* magazine by day and mixing cocktails in a trendy Soho bar by night to pay the rent; that was on top of her late night at the Blast launch, which had indeed turned out to be a blast. But she, too, had an important date pending. Adam, the complete sweetie, had put in a good word for her with Astrid, fashion guru at Aristo PR for the assistant's job. Jaz had offered her services faster than you can say 'mood-boosting bracelet' and an interview had been set up.

'No pizza for me, thanks,' said Kate, who was sporting a face-pack and a fetching flowery shower cap (having just applied a deep-conditioning treatment to her new power bob). Tomorrow she wanted to shine – and not just on the career front.
'It's unlike you to turn down carbohydrate, Kate,' said Chrissie, smiling sweetly and flicking back her long, blonde hair. Kate gritted her teeth.
'How much longer is Chrissie going to be living under the same roof?', she wondered. Out loud, she said:

'I wish you wouldn't make such a mess during your temporary stay here, Chrissie.' It was water off a duck's back. Chrissie, to Kate's great annoyance, had taken to performing a nightly one-woman fashion show as she tried to decide what to wear to work the next day. She was loving her new job at Devastation Records. She had to compete with the Damien Hirst fish tank in reception for attention, but she was certain she'd be 'discovered', even if it did mean getting up an hour earlier than she would have liked to do her hair and make-up in the mornings.

Chrissie was planning a special effort for tomorrow's date with Steve. True, it was Laura who Steve was interested in – Chrissie's (blind) date was supposedly Steve's old school friend. But she was planning to win Steve's undivided attention by the end of the first course. After all, Laura, wearing her TV researcher's uniform of combats and trainers, was no match.

But Chrissie almost dropped her slice of pizza when Laura picked up a pink slingback from under the table and asked to borrow it. Laura didn't give two hoots about tomorrow's date. As far as she was concerned, Steve was ghastly. Anyway, she only had eyes for John, the elusive assistant producer. She'd agreed to go on this date partly because she was a clever networker who rarely turned down invitations, but also because she was planning to trial-run a whole new look (Chrissie and Jaz must be getting to her).

'So, Pol, what are you up to tomorrow?' asked Kate. 'Oh, nothing much. Harry's out with the boys so I'll probably watch TV,' was the reply. Secretly, Polly was very excited. Simon had phoned that afternoon to say that he would be in London for the weekend and had invited her to dinner. Needless to say, she had already booked a manicure and leg wax, and a blow-dry with Charles for Saturday morning.

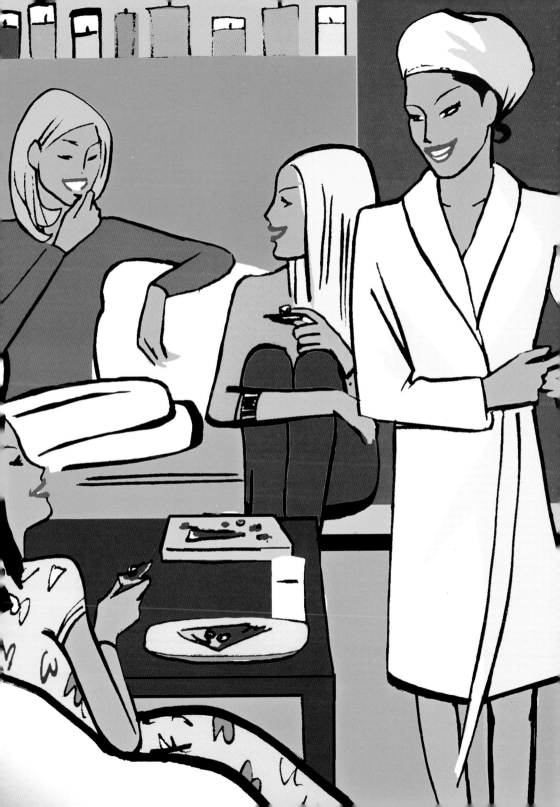

praise the up-do

Whether it's a simple top knot or a polished French pleat, an updo can make you feel really pulled together and glamorous. Putting your hair up can give you a big confidence boost. Not only is it an instant fix for a bad-hair day, but if you are going out after work, an updo can help you to switch instantly into out-to-play mode. And don't think that putting your hair up is only for formal events. Björk-style twists and scrunched-up top knots are great for clubs and hot, sweaty atmospheres. (It's one way to ensure that your hair stays up as long as you do!) If it's a really big date, nothing beats going to the salon to have your hair put up professionally. But even at home, mastering the art of the updo is a cinch.

the high pony

Ponytails, worn high on the head, Versace-style, can look great for evening. The effect can be super-sexy, rather than sweet and innocent. An added advantage is that a high, tight ponytail is renowned for its instant face-lifting effects. This style works best on unwashed hair because it is easier to work with.

you need
Smoothing brush • covered elastic band or piece of wet string • matt hair grip • serum or glossing spray

1 For a sleek look, brush your hair, pull it back and fix it on top of your crown with a covered elastic band. Alternatively, use a wet piece of string, which will contract as it dries, holding the hair in place securely.

2 Cover the band with a scarf or take a piece of hair from the ponytail, wrap it around the band and secure it underneath with a matt hair grip.

3 Smooth the hair with serum or glossing spray.

the chignon

Chignons – as worn by Audrey Hepburn, Eva Perón and Grace Kelly – are just *so* chic. They're also a great way to look groomed on a bad hair day.

you need
Gel or hairspray • a covered elastic band or a piece of string • matt hair grips • a hairnet if your hair is layered • serum

1 Apply a little gel or hairspray to smooth back the hair and sweep it into a ponytail at the nape.

2 Twist the hair around the elastic band or string as if making a figure-of-eight shape to create a neat bun.

3 Fasten with grips and cover with a hairnet to keep the ends neat. Or leave off the hairnet and pull a few strands forward to soften the look.

4 Smooth a couple of drops of serum over the surface for extra shine.

french pleat

Arguably the the most elegant way to put your hair up – think of Catherine Deneuve's neat French pleat in the film *Belle du Jour*.

you need
Medium or firm setting lotion • hairdryer • matt hair grips • hairspray

1 Set or blow-dry your hair loosely, using a medium or firm setting lotion. (Continued on page 63.)

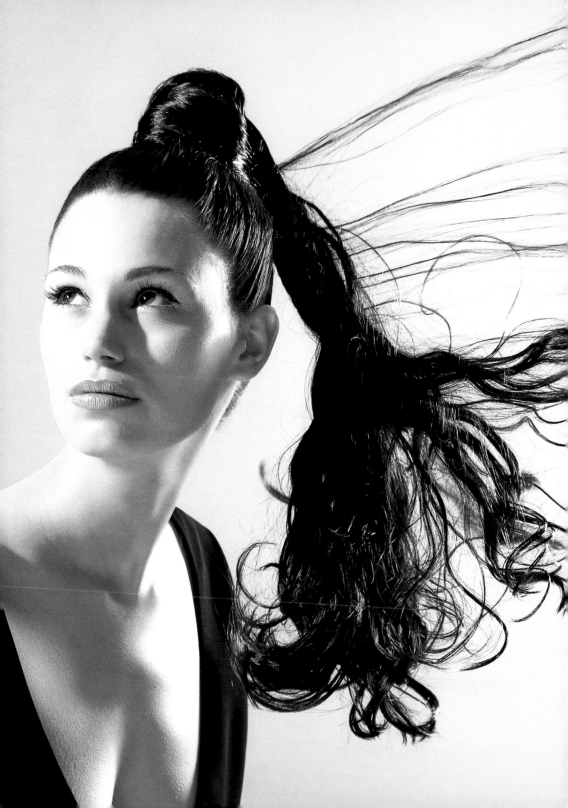

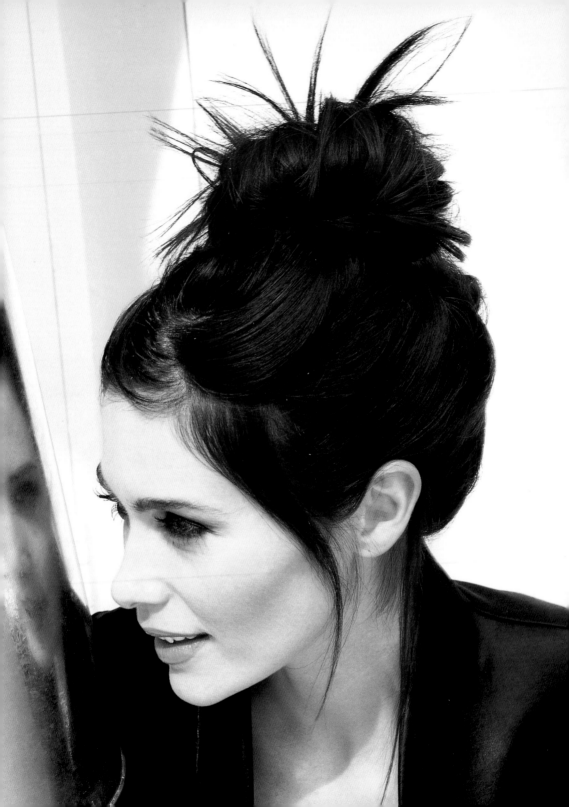

2 Gently run your fingers through your hair to break it up.

3 Twist the hair up the back of the head and, holding it tightly, secure it in place using matt hair grips.

4 Spray the hair with hairspray to hold the style in place.

5 For a modern take on the classic French pleat, splay out a few ends from the top section to give the style a slightly dishevelled finish (left).

spiky twists

This funky hairstyle works best on medium-length hair. It is a great look for clubbing and parties and is actually a lot easier to do than it appears. Make sure, though, that this style complements the shape of your head and face.

you need
Comb • strong-hold hairspray • matt hair grips

1 Gently backcomb the hair and spritz it all over with a strong-hold hairspray.

2 Take random sections of hair, about 4 sq cm (1½ sq in) in size, and twist them tightly from the base to the ends. Keep twisting each section until it coils back against the scalp, forming a top-knot.

3 Using matt hair grips, pin the twists securely against the head, allowing the ends to work themselves loose to create a spiky effect. It's a good idea to cross the grips as this will give maximum support and hold.

4 Continue in this way until the whole head is covered with top-knots.

5 Gently tease and splay out the ends of the hair to create a spiky effect (see right).

top-knot scrunchies

This is a similar style to the Spiky Twists but the end result is a head full of neat little top-knots.

you need
Comb • strong-hold hairspray • matt hair grips • firm-hold wax

1 Follow steps 1 and 2 for spiky twists.

2 Secure the top-knots firmly to the scalp using matt hair grips as before, but make sure that the ends of the hair are neatly tucked under.

3 To finish, apply a little firm-hold wax to each scrunchie to smooth down any stray hairs.

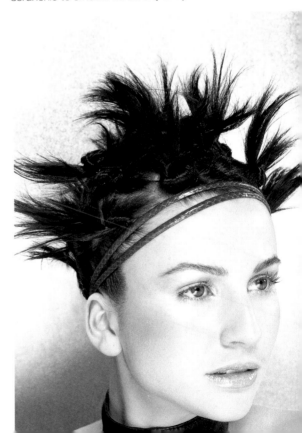

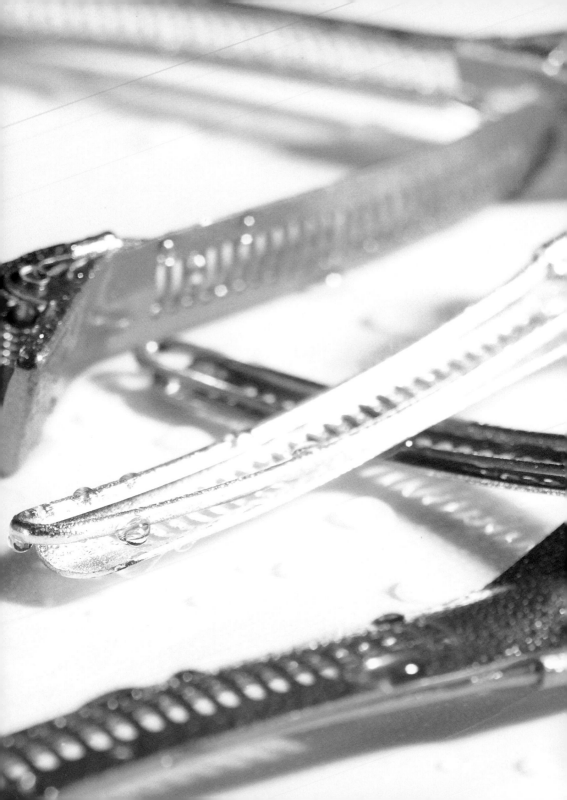

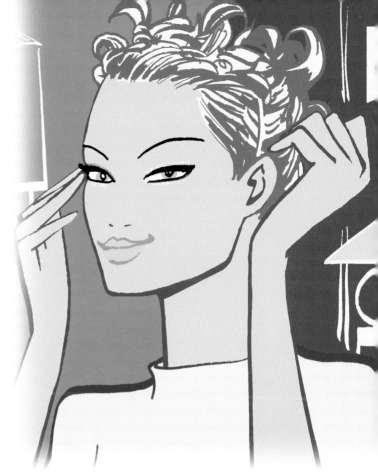

... polly tries a funky updo

Polly leaves the girls downstairs and retreats to her boudoir for a bit of peace. She sits down in front of her dressing-table and tries out some of Jaz's new glittery eyeshadow in preparation for her date on Saturday. (Jaz, in true form, had left her make-up strewn all over the bathroom.) She's dying to tell the other girls about sexy cyber-suitor Simon and their little snog in New York, but she knows it isn't a good idea. She feels so guilty about Harry and anyway, Jaz and

Chrissie are terrible at keeping secrets. Still, she tells herself, there's no harm in having dinner with Simon as he passes through town en route to Geneva. The eyeshadow looks somewhat out of place with her layered, shoulder-length blonde hair. Polly feels like throwing caution to the wind. After all, on Saturday she'll be off-duty and for once not wearing one of her neat little suits. Absentmindedly, she twists a section of hair around her finger and pins it to the

crown of her head (as seen in one of Jaz's copies of *Gloss*). The effect is very funky and very un-Polly, but she rather likes it. She carries on twisting random sections of hair, allowing the ends to work themselves loose, creating a spiky effect. By the time she's finished, the effect is more funky urban chick than frumpy City banker. The added advantage is that if she bumps into anyone she knows on her illicit date, they almost certainly won't recognize her.

updo dos
and don'ts

DON'T try and put up newly washed hair as it is just too slippery and floppy to handle.

DO soften a chignon or bun by loosening some wisps of hair around the face, otherwise the overall effect can appear a bit harsh.

DON'T try anything too complicated or too structured so that it looks as though you've tried too hard. (Ivana Trump's beehive is not the look to aim for!)

DON'T use hairpieces for the first time on a big date. It's best to experiment with them beforehand. Your hairdo slipping into your soup is not going to make a good impression.

DO remember to backcomb the roots of your hair. This will set a firm foundation for the perfect updo.

DO use accessories. They are perfect as a quick cover-up for a not-so-perfect updo.

DO use coloured mascaras to brighten up selected pieces of hair.

DO carry a handbag-size can of hairspray and some matt hair grips with you at all times to rescue your updo in an emergency.

DO use an invisible hairnet around a bun to keep the hair in place, especially if your hair is layered or has straggly ends.

DON'T try too hard. Sometimes the quickest and messiest updos look the best.

DON'T use accessories that are too heavy as they will pull down an updo and ruin the look.

DO make the most of long hair if you have it. There are times when bigger is definitely better.

HAIR SNIP
FOR SALON-STYLE HAIR AT HOME IN AN INSTANT: TO MAKE LONG HAIR LOOK FABULOUS IN NO TIME AT ALL, HERE IS A QUICK, SIMPLE HAIR-UP TRICK. SECURE THE HAIR IN A PONYTAIL HIGH ON THE CROWN USING A COVERED ELASTIC BAND. AS YOU PULL THE PONYTAIL THROUGH, CATCH THE ENDS IN THE BAND TO FORM A LOOP. ARRANGE THE ENDS INTO A FAN SHAPE AND SEPARATE THEM WITH GEL. IT DOESN'T MATTER IF THE STRANDS WORK THEMSELVES LOOSE, THIS ONLY ENHANCES THE LOOK.

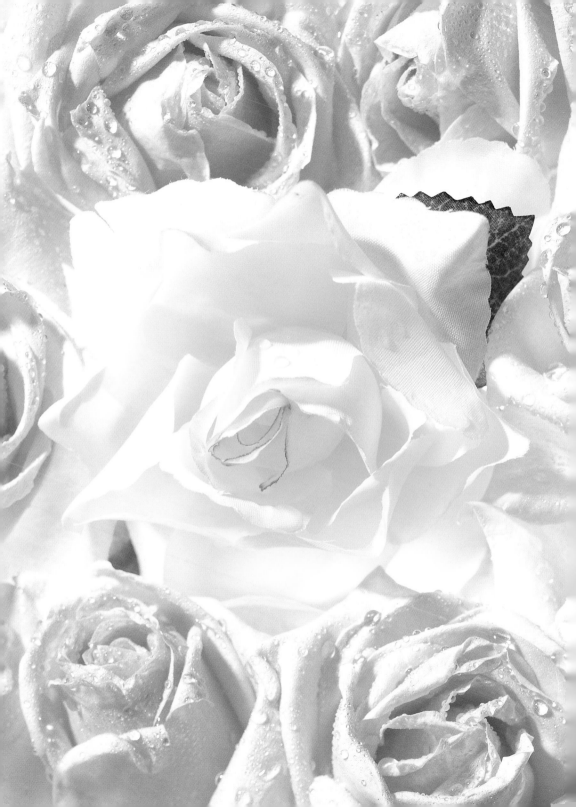

corn-rows

This is a very groovy look, but be warned: you need to have an elegantly shaped head as this can be quite severe. If you want to try this style for the first time, it's a good idea to go to a salon and have it done professionally, but if you are good at plaiting, try doing it using the following instructions.

you need

Comb • sectioning clips • snag-free mini elastics (coloured bands or hair beads, optional) • matt hair grips

1 Section the hair into lots of small 'rows' from the forehead to the nape, holding them out of the way with sectioning clips.

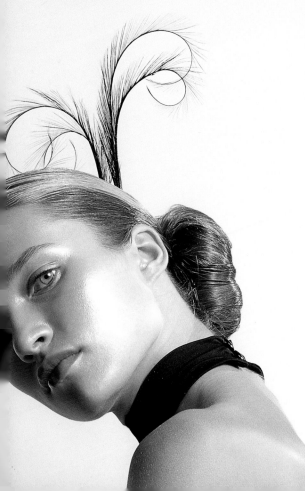

2 Starting at the forehead, plait each section into a mini French plait, keeping them tight against the scalp.

3 Secure each plait with a mini elastic band. Different coloured bands or beads can be used for a quirky effect.

4 If you find it too difficult to plait, just twist each section tightly instead and secure it using matt hair grips.

bun rings

A speedy, easy way to put long hair up is to use a bun ring (you'll find them in most large pharmacies).

you need
Smoothing brush • snag-free elastic band • hairspray • bun ring • matt hair grips • tail comb • light glossing spray

1 Using a smoothing brush, scrape your hair back into a low ponytail, securing it at the nape with a snag-free band. Spray hairspray onto a huge make-up brush and smooth it over the surface of the hair to control any stray ends.

2 Place a bun ring around the ponytail and secure it with matt hair grips.

3 Start to wrap the hair around the bun ring section by section, and secure it with matt hair grips.

4 Carry on until you have completely covered the bun ring and all the sections are neatly secured in place.

5 When the hair is secure, gently pull a few wispy strands out of the bun using the end of the tail comb and finish by spraying with a light glossing spray (right).

6 Stick a feather or decorative hairpin through the bun if you want to add drama (left).

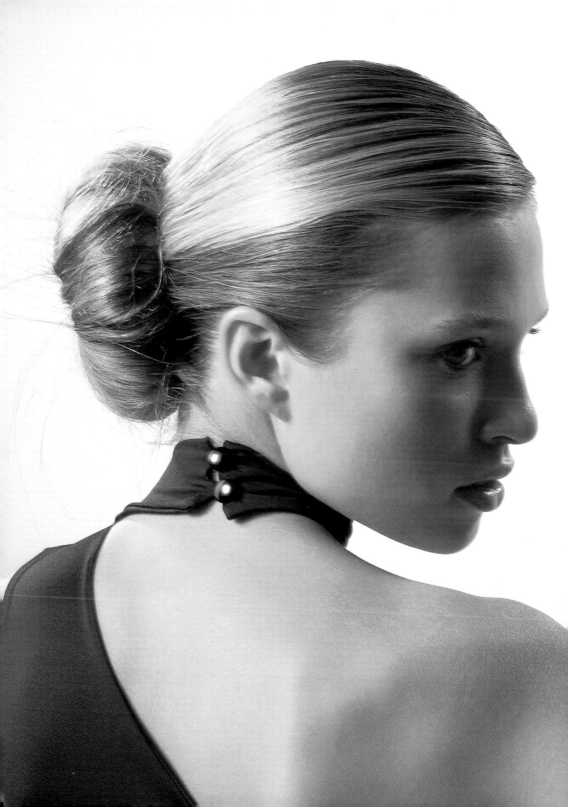

fake an updo

Even if your hair is only medium-length or shorter, it is still possible to create an impressive up-sweep by weaving a little practical magic with a hairpiece.

mane piece

The foolproof way to secure a hairpiece is to take a 2-cm (¾-in) section of your own hair at the crown or below. Twist it into a knot and pin it. Then place the comb of the hairpiece into the knot and pin it on either side. For a really slick finish, try the following.

you need

Snag-free elastic • matt hair grips • weft of hair approximately 1 m (3.2 ft) long • fine hairpin

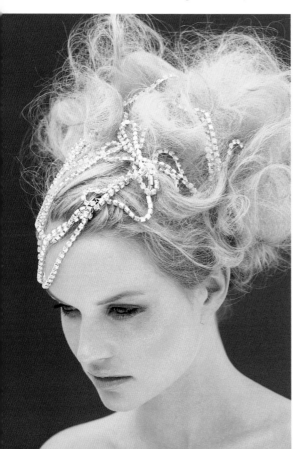

1 Sweep your hair back into a tight ponytail at the nape and secure it with a snag-free elastic.

2 Attach the weft of hair, wrapping it once around the base of your ponytail and securing it with matt hair grips.

3 Take a small section of the weft and wrap it around the ponytail a few times to disguise the join and secure it underneath with a fine hairpin.

uptown girl

This is a look that is guaranteed to turn a few heads.

you need

Hot rollers • hairspray • bun ring • matt hair grips • hairbrush • long diamanté necklace (optional) • hairpins

1 Set your hair on large hot rollers and lightly spritz it with hairspray.

2 When the rollers are cool, take them out and let the curls droop slightly.

3 Pile the hair through a bun ring and use matt hair grips to hold it in place.

4 Backbrush the hair loosely, causing it to 'candy floss'.

5 Sweep and swirl the hair randomly around the head, allowing tendrils to fall across the face and making sure to retain some height on the crown and conceal the bun ring (right).

6 If you want to accessorize, push the hair back and drape a diamanté necklace over the front of the hair, securing it with hairpins (left).

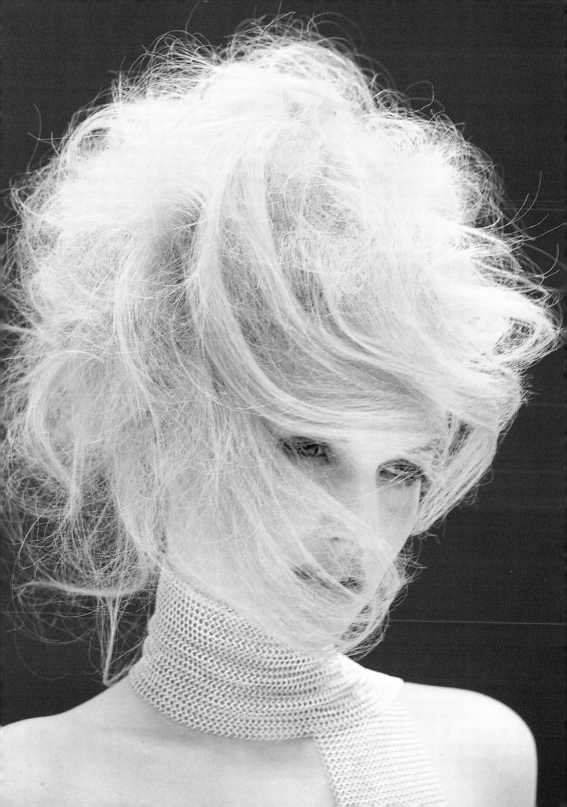

dressing updos

Accessories and hair make-up are just as effective for adorning an updo as they are for dressing up loose hair. Everything from glitter slides and beaded hair grips to feathered combs and a diamanté tiara can add drama and glamour to even the most understated chignon, pleat or twist. An updo, however, does open up new accessorizing opportunities: beaded hairpins, decorative chopsticks and feathers are all winners.

stencilling

To add even more oomph to an updo for a big night out, try the following stencilling technique.

you need

Stencil • washable body paint • narrow paintbrush • glitter powder • hairspray

HAIR SNIP

ALWAYS CHOOSE YOUR ACCESSORIES TO MATCH YOUR OUTFIT AND YOUR MOOD. IF IT'S A BIG NIGHT OUT, GO BIG, USING FLOWERS – EITHER REAL OR FAKE – FEATHERS AND COLOURFUL BEADS. IF YOU JUST WANT TO BRIGHTEN UP A DULL OUTFIT, GO SMALLER AND MORE UNDERSTATED.

CHOOSE STURDY ACCESSORIES THAT ARE TOTALLY SEALED AT THE ENDS. THERE IS NOTHING WORSE THAN A GLITZY ACCESSORY BREAKING HALFWAY THROUGH THE NIGHT, OR NOT BEING ABLE TO REMOVE ONE AT THE END OF IT.

1 Choose your stencil design to work with your overall look. You can either buy a pre-cut stencil from a home-decorating store or make your own by drawing or tracing your design onto a piece of stiff paper and cut it out with a craft knife.

2 Position the stencil on the hair and gently dab on the paint with the brush until you have filled in the design. Then dab a little glitter powder onto the wet paint. Make sure you hold the stencil very still to avoid any smudging or a blurred outline.

3 Carefully remove the stencil and blast with hairspray to set the design (see page 75).

it's a wrap

Ribbons and cords look stunning wrapped around an updo, but you do need a lot of height.

you need

Hairdryer • blow-drying spray • comb • hairspray • matt hair grips • cord

1 Roughly dry the hair using a blow-drying spray, which is ideal as it is not too heavy.

2 Tip your head upside-down, letting all the hair fall forwards. Lightly backcomb the hair to give it volume and spray it with hairspray.

3 Use a matt hair grip to attach the end of the cord to the hair at the nape, then start wrapping it around the backcombed section. You will get a better hold if you do this randomly.

4 Tie the cord around the top section of the hair and secure it with a grip (see page 76).

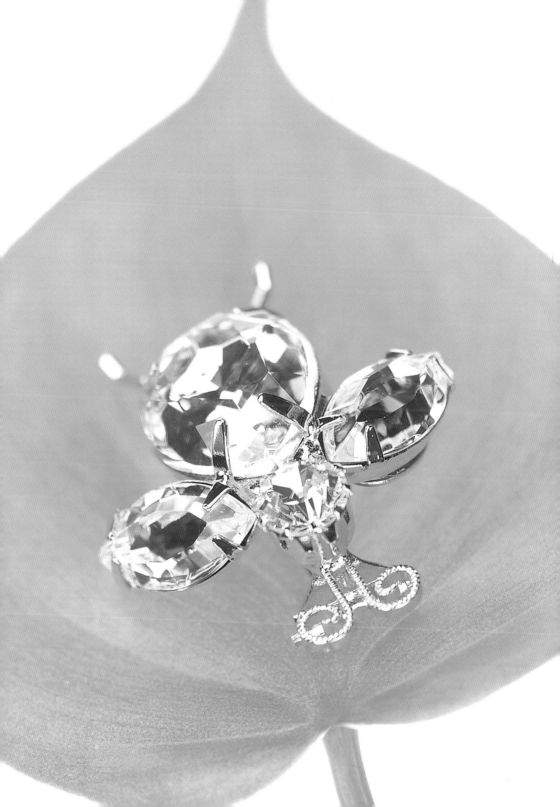

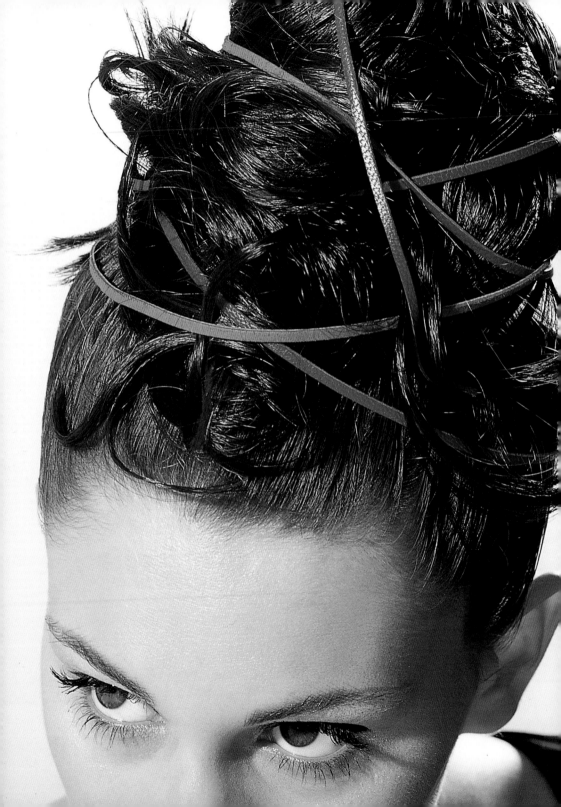

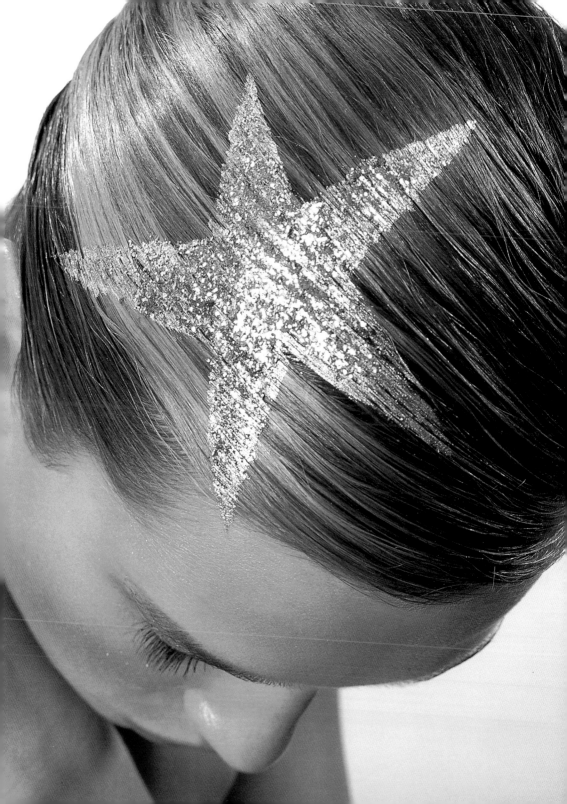

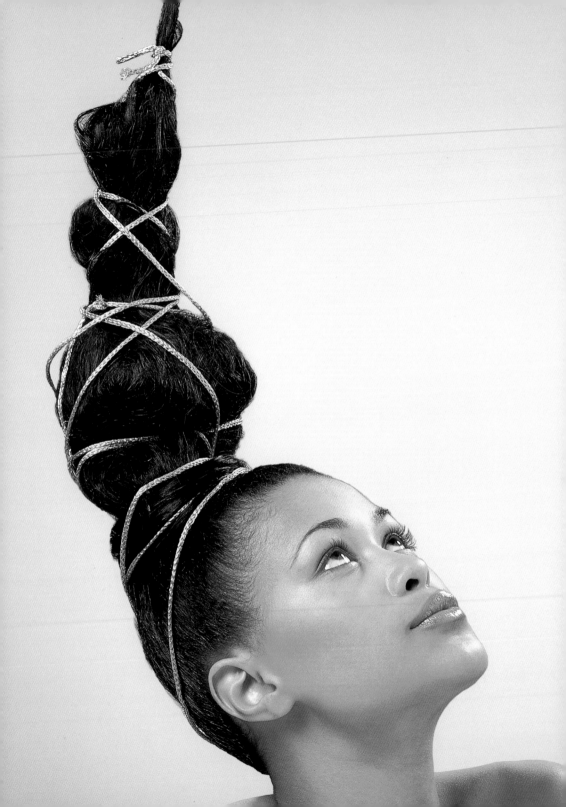

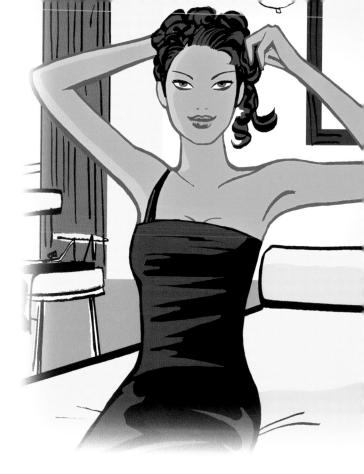

Kate kicks off her power heel with relief and collapses onto the hideously patterned hotel bedspread. God, playing the

... kate does day-into-night hair

part of Miss-Get-Ahead-At-Work is so exhausting. It's 7 pm and the conference has only just finished. Several times during the day's coffee breaks, she had tried to get Matthew to listen to her idea for marketing the new low-fat biscuit brand, but to no avail. All he was interested in was whether she had managed to take down all the minutes. Oh well, there's always this evening to further her career ... Damn, is that really the time?

She's got less than half an hour to get ready. Preparing to jump in the shower, Kate pulls her hair swiftly into a ponytail, catching the ends in a covered elastic band to form a casual updo. Glancing in the mirror, she realizes that her emergency shower-do actually looks quite good. It's just as well, as she doesn't have enough time to wash her hair and wear it down – it would take hours to preen all those unruly curls into some

sort of shape. Feeling refreshed and revived from the shower, she climbs into her slinky black evening dress (her favourite floral dresses were just too country bumpkin to cut it on the career front, she's decided). Spiking out the ends of her impromptu updo, she pulls a few strands of hair around her face free to soften the final effect and dabs on some glitter gel. Kate is ready to be the belle of the Crunch ball.

... big date night

'**Come on, Laura** ... it's 8 o'clock and we're late,' yelled Chrissie, pacing up and down the hallway. She looked fabulously lean and willowy in her silvery sequinned jeans and black halterneck top, her hair pulled into a high, Versace-style ponytail. The girls had arranged to meet at home and then take a minicab into town for their double date. But what was Laura up to? She never took longer than ten minutes to get ready, while Chrissie usually took two hours. 'She's probably doing sit-ups or something,' thought Chrissie, knowing Laura's passion for working out.

'I'm coming,' replied Laura, as she negotiated her way down the stairs in Chrissie's elegant pink sling-backs. Chrissie swayed on her stiletto spikes. In place of the usual combats, Laura was wearing a scarlet skirt embroidered with flowers and a stretchy pink top. Her hair looked softer and more flirty than usual and she had little rosebuds clipped into it.
'Wow,' said Chrissie, somewhat taken aback (and, if truth be known, rather piqued) by the unexpected competition. She had never seen Laura looking this good. 'Oh, by the way, Steve phoned earlier to change the venue to Cirque instead of Rush.' Laura shrugged her shoulders as she wondered if Steve's friend could possibly be as dreadful as Steve.

Meanwhile, over at the offices of Bartrum Inc. Bank, Polly was in a panic. Simon had arrived from New York a day early and had called that morning to ask if she could make dinner this evening. She should have said no. Instead, she'd rushed out at lunchtime to buy a new slinky black dress (well, what were bonuses for?). Now she was in the bathroom getting ready. She hadn't had time to wash her hair this morning, thanks to Chrissie hogging the bathroom. So she resorted to her favourite bad-hair-day fix and pulled her blonde hair back into a sleek chignon. Five minutes later she was hailing a cab in the street outside, 'Can you take me to Cirque, please?'

Chrissie stalked into the downstairs bar at Cirque, followed closely by Laura who, for someone more used to wearing trainers, had gained command of her kitten heels remarkably quickly. Steve was waiting at the bar alone, wearing leather jeans, a fake tan and a smug expression. 'Well, hello girls,' he practically drooled over Laura.
'Where's your friend?' asked Chrissie, sharply. She wasn't going to be able to divert his attention away from Laura if there were only three of them.
'Right behind you.' Laura looked over her shoulder and practically fell over.

Standing behind them was ... John – the object of Laura's desire. Yep, Steve's single friend and Chrissie's blind date was none other than gorgeous, sexy, elusive assistant TV producer, John.

Upstairs, Polly walked through the door of Cirque, her heart pounding – she wasn't sure whether it was passion or guilt, but she certainly hoped she wouldn't bump into any of Harry's friends. She could already see Simon, waiting patiently at a corner table. He looked heart-stoppingly gorgeous. Aaggh! What would they talk about? He hadn't mentioned their little tryst in his e-mails – maybe he'd gone off her? Polly still wasn't sure if the tone of this dinner was to be work or pleasure.

Chrissie, meanwhile, was losing patience. Steve wasn't paying her enough attention. Still, Cirque seemed to be packed with good-looking men. 'Time to go walkabout,' she thought. 'Perhaps to the ladies loo upstairs to fix my lipstick.' Swinging her slim hips through the restaurant doors, she suddenly saw a very familiar face. It couldn't be – yes, it was. Polly was sitting opposite a completely lush man who looked devastatingly attentive as he kissed her hand. 'Polly,' said Chrissie eyeing up Simon suspiciously, 'what are you doing here?'